Proceedings

Volume 600

Progress in Holographic Applications

Jean Ebbeni
Chairman/Editor

Organized by
SPIE—The International Society for Optical Engineering
ANRT—Association Nationale de la Recherche Technique

5-6 December 1985
Cannes, France

Published by
SPIE—The International Society for Optical Engineering
P.O. Box 10, Bellingham, Washington 98227-0010 USA
Telephone 206/676-3290 (Pacific Time) • Telex 46-7053

SPIE (The Society of Photo-Optical Instrumentation Engineers) is a nonprofit society dedicated to advancing engineering
and scientific applications of optical, electro-optical, and optoelectronic instrumentation, systems, and technology.

mw 3-31-87

The papers appearing in this book comprise the proceedings of the meeting mentioned on the cover and title page. They reflect the authors' opinions and are published as presented and without change, in the interests of timely dissemination. Their inclusion in this publication does not necessarily constitute endorsement by the editors or by SPIE.

Please use the following format to cite material from this book:
    Author(s), "Title of Paper," *Progress in Holographic Applications*, Jean Ebbeni, Editor, Proc. SPIE 600, page numbers (1986).

Library of Congress Catalog Card No. 85-063818
ISBN 0-89252-635-1

Printed in the United States of America.

PROGRESS IN HOLOGRAPHIC APPLICATIONS

Volume 600

Contents

Conference 600, Progress in Holographic Applications was one of eighteen technical conferences presented at the

2nd International Technical Symposium on
Optical and Electro-Optical Applied Science and Engineering
Palais des Festivals et des Congrès • Cannes, France • 25 November-6 December 1985

Cooperating Sponsors

American Society of Photogrammetry
ANRT—Association Nationale de la Recherche Technique
Associazione Elettrotecnica ed Elettronica Italiana
Austrian Physical Society
Battelle-Geneva Research Centres
British Computer Society
British Pattern Recognition Association
CNES—Centre National d'Etudes Spatiales
Comité Belge d'Optique
DGaO—Deutsche Gesellschaft für angewandte Optik
Ecole Polytechnique Fédérale de Lausanne
EFOMP—European Federation of Organisations for Medical Physics
Eurographics—The European Association for Computer Graphics
European Association for Signal Processing
European Space Agency
IEEE Computer Society

Information Processing Society of Japan
IFIP—International Federation for Information Processing
Israel Laser and Electro-Optics Society
Jet Propulsion Laboratory/California Institute of Technology
NASA—National Aeronautics and Space Administration
Optical Engineering Society of China
Optics Division of the European Physical Society
SGOEM—Schweizerische Gesellschaft für Optik und Elektronenmikroskopie
Sira Ltd.—The Research Association for Instrumentation
SEE—Société des Electriciens, des Electroniciens et des Radioélectriciens
SGOIP—Syndicat Général de l'Optique et des Instruments de Précision
Société Française d'Optique
Society for Information Display
Society of Photographic Scientists and Engineers
SPIE—The International Society for Optical Engineering

Technical Organizing Committee

Raymond Ackaouy (France)
Hervé J. Arditty** (France)
Lionel R. Baker (UK)
H. Bauch (West Germany)
J. Besson (France)
J. A. M. Bleeker (Netherlands)
Robert Boirat (France)
Rémy Bouillie (France)
C. Braccini (Italy)
H. J. Caulfield (USA)
P. Chavel (France)
B. Chen (USA)
A. M. Coblentz (France)
E. le Coquil (France)
Francis J. Corbett (USA)
J. L. Culhane (UK)
I. Debusschère (Belgium)
Gilbert J. Declerck (Belgium)
Th. deGraauw (Netherlands)
Michael J. B. Duff (UK)
Jean Ebbeni (Belgium)
R. Edgar (UK)
C. T. Elliott (UK)
P. Encrenaz (France)
Reiner Esselborn (West Germany)
William F. Fagan** (West Germany)
Olivier D. Faugeras (France)
Armin Felske (West Germany)
Robert E. Fischer** (USA)
G. I. Frank (Canada)
D. J. le Gall (France)
G. Giralt (France)
P. Goldsmith (USA)
G. H. Granlund (Sweden)
Karl H. Guenther (Liechtenstein)
D. Hardy (France)
A. Hartog (UK)
J. P. Haton (France)
E. Heijne (Switzerland)
Robin E. Herron (USA)
B. Hok (Sweden)
R. J. Horne (UK)
T. S. Huang (USA)

J. P. Huignard (France)
K. Inada (Japan)
C. Jaffe (USA)
J. Jerphagnon (France)
Luc B. Jeunhomme (France)
P. Kammenos (France)
Ke Jing Tang (China)
Robert Kelley (USA)
R. Kist (West Germany)
Lydie Koch-Miramond (France)
Eric Kollberg (Sweden)
O. Kübler (Switzerland)
Murat Kunt (Switzerland)
P. Kuttner (West Germany)
J. C. LaTombe (France)
John W. Lear (USA)
Maurice LeLuyer (France)
William Lenne (France)
H. Maître (France)
André Masson (France)
K. Matsumoto (Japan)
Alain Mellah (France)
John Melles (Netherlands)
M. Mercier (France)
John Midwinter (UK)
A. Moncalvo (Italy)
André Monfils (Belgium)
Michel Monnerie (France)
F. D. Morten (UK)
Gaylord E. Moss (USA)
M. Murata (Japan)
H. G. Mussman (West Germany)
T. Nakayama (Japan)
E. Naeumann (West Germany)
H. H. Nagel (West Germany)
Yoshio Nakamura (Japan)
Jean-Pierre Noblanc (France)
André Oosterlinck (Belgium)
O. Parriaux (Switzerland)
P. Paulet (France)
Thomas Pearsall (USA)
D. Pearson (UK)
N. J. Phillips (UK)

Roy F. Potter (USA)
E. Reinhardt (West Germany)
S. C. Rashleigh (Australia)
F. Rocca (Italy)
H. P. Roeser (West Germany)
P. J. Rogers (UK)
Sidney L. Russak (USA)
D. Rutovitz (UK)
N. Saks (USA)
A. M. Scheggi (Italy)
H. Schnopper (Denmark)
John S. Seeley** (UK)
J. Shamir (Israel)
Howard J. Siegel (USA)
J. Simon (France)
Siv Cheng Tang (France)
P. Smigielski (France)
R. W. Sparrow (UK)
Irving Spiro (USA)
H. Steinbichler (West Germany)
P. Stewart (UK)
Paul Suetens (Belgium)
B. G. Taylor (Netherlands)
Andrew G. Tescher* (USA)
C. J. Todd (USA)
Brian A. Tozer (UK)
J. L. Tribillon (France)
J. D. Trolinger (USA)
J. Trumper (West Germany)
J. Tsujiuchi (Japan)
J. Vermeiren (Belgium)
B. Vowinkel (West Germany)
Peter Waddell (UK)
G. Watkins (USA)
B. M. Watrasiewicz (UK)
T. L. Williams (UK)
Ingo Wilmanns (West Germany)
R. G. Wilson (UK)
Myron W. Wolbarsht (USA)
W. Wolfe (USA)
B. Woodcock (UK)
G. T. Wrixon (UK)
Joseph Yaver (USA)
I. T. Young (Netherlands)
Pierre Zaleski (France)
P. Zamperoni (West Germany)

International Technical Advisory Committee

Nils Abramson (Sweden)
Leo Beckmann (Netherlands)
Julian Bescos (Spain)
James B. Breckinridge (USA)
Jean Bulabois (France)
Jean Ebbeni (Belgium)
Hedzer A. Ferwerda (Netherlands)
Hans J. Frankena (Netherlands)
Jean Gay (France)
Joseph W. Goodman (USA)
Goesta H. Granlund (Sweden)
Daniel M. Gross (Switzerland)
Cyril Hilsum (UK)
Harold H. Hopkins (UK)
Christian Imbert (France)
Erik Ingelstam (Sweden)
Roland Jacobsson (Sweden)
Ralf Th. Kersten (West Germany)
A. Labeyrie (France)
Jean-Pierre Laude (France)
Lewis Larmore (USA)
Serge Lowenthal (France)
André Maréchal (France)
Ernst Mathieu (Switzerland)
Brian L. Morgan (UK)
Gerhard J. Müller (West Germany)
Henk Olthof (France)
Daniel B. Ostrowsky (France)
Philippe Robert (Switzerland)
Rainer Röhler (West Germany)
A. M. Scheggi (Italy)
Dieter Schuöcker (Austria)
Joseph Shamir (Israel)
Warren J. Smith (USA)
O. D. D. Soares (Portugal)
Alberto Sona (Italy)
Erich Spitz (France)
Brian J. Thompson (USA)
Hans Tiziani (West Germany)
Reinhard Ulrich (West Germany)
Hermann Walter (West Germany)
Vivian K. Walworth (USA)
Roy Welch (USA)
James C. Wyant (USA)
Charles L. Wyman (USA)

*Chairman of Technical Organizing Committee
**Vice-Chairmen of Technical Organizing Committee

PROGRESS IN HOLOGRAPHIC APPLICATIONS

Volume 600

Conference Committee

Chairman: **Jean Ebbeni,** Université Libre de Bruxelles, Belgium
Co-Chairman: **Gaylord E. Moss,** Hughes Aircraft Company, USA

Program Committee
H. J. Caulfield, Aerodyne Research Incorporated, USA; **J. P. Huignard,** Thomson CSF, France; **K. Matsumoto,** Canon Incorporated, Japan; **N. J. Phillips,** Loughborough University of Technology, United Kingdom; **J. L. Tribillon,** Holo-Laser, France; **J. Tsujiuchi,** Tokyo Institute of Technology, Japan; **B. Woodcock,** Pilkington P.E. Ltd., United Kingdom

Session Chairmen
Session 1—New Holographic Materials, **Jean Ebbeni,** Université Libre de Bruxelles, Belgium; **N. J. Phillips,** Loughborough University of Technology, United Kingdom
Session 2—Holographic Optical Elements, **J. L. Tribillon,** Holo-Laser, France; **K. Matsumoto,** Canon Incorporated, Japan
Session 3—Multiplexing in Holography, **J. P. Huignard,** Thomson CSF, France; **B. Woodcock,** Pilkington P.E. Ltd., United Kingdom
Session 4—Special Techniques, **Gaylord E. Moss,** Hughes Aircraft Company, USA; **H. J. Caulfield,** Aerodyne Research Incorporated, USA

INTRODUCTION

Holography is a powerful technique which is very useful in an enormous range of applications, from artistic expression to the most sophisticated measurements of external fields. Some uses, such as holographic interferometry, are well known. However, other developments are rapidly emerging and are emphasized in these Proceedings.

Holographic optical elements are being introduced into systems because of their compactness and low cost as well as for their performance of functions that are not possible with conventional reflective or refractive elements. Some new materials for the optical elements are described, such as photopolymers, which require shorter exposure time and reduced processing complexity and also possess an increased environmental stability.

Several papers describing state-of-the-art techniques in general applications related to holography show the rapid rise of development in this field. Different holographic multiplex techniques are described for telecommunications applications.

Jean Ebbeni
Université Libre de Bruxelles, Belgium

PROGRESS IN HOLOGRAPHIC APPLICATIONS

Volume 600

Session 1

New Holographic Materials

Chairmen
Jean Ebbeni
Université Libre de Bruxelles, Belgium

N. J. Phillips
Loughborough University of Technology, United Kingdom

General Review on Recording Materials used in Holography

Jean-Louis   TRIBILLON

Research and Development, Holo - Laser
12, rue de Vouillé - 75015 Paris - FRANCE

Abstract

An ideal material for the application of holography would be defined as a material that has a sensitivity suited to existing lasers, a high resolution, a linear transfer function, and a low noise ; it is also indefinetely recyclable, and it is relatively cheap. Numerous efforts have been made to produce this sort of material. We examine the principal recording materials used in holography that now exist.

Introduction

Since holography exists, the question is : which recording material ?
The ideal recording material could be defined as follows :
- it has a sensitivity well suited to existing lasers,
- it has a high resolution in order to record interference fringes,
- its transfer function is linear in order to reproduce a good image of the object,
- it has a low noise,
- it is relatively cheap,
- it can be indefinetely recycled,

Today, after 20 years, this material does not exist.

However, an important effort is made in setting up a material better suited to holography.

Actually, the question, today, is not which recording material for holography but which material for which holographic application ? The application will therefore determine the material.

Thus it should not be suprising that today some materials are better suited for holographic non-destructive test, for 3-D display, for holographic optical elements (silver halide and dichromated gelatin, thermoplastics,...) that others already available or soon available are going to respond to new needs such as mass produced holographic optical elements, optical information processing, computer generated holograms (photoresists, photopolymers, electro-optical crystals, for example).

It is therefore interesting to rapidly investigate these materials, since the development of holographic applications and recording materials for holography are interdependant.

The silver halide emulsions

It's an "old material" but considerable improvements have been made on this type of material in recent years. Of course it is mainly the extension of techniques used for photographic emulsions   (1).

An holographic plate is similar to a photographic plate, only the values of some characteristic features are modified in order to satisfy holographic needs :
- the silver halide grains are extremely thin in order to record high spatial frequencies,
- since holography deals with lasers, they are made sensitive to each type of laser.

Characteristic features of silver halide emulsions :
- energetic sensitivity :
This material is one of the most sensitive : 1 to 100 $\mu J/cm^2$
- spectral sensitivity :
Holographic plates are made sensitive, selectively, to each type of laser (blue, green, red).
- resolution
It mainly depends on the dimension of the grains in emulsion. The important improvements made in recent years (Agfa-Gevaert has improved the average dimension of the grain from 50 nm (8E56 plate) to 35 nm (8E56HD plate) offering to the users plates that can resolve several thousand lines per mm.
- frequency response :
An illumination implies not only transparency variation but also thickness and index variations of the gelatin. It is therefore necessary to analyse the response following two components :
  magnitude response and phase response.
* Modulation Transfer Function (M T F) :
Current modulation transfer function holographic plates keep more than 80 % of the fringes contrast for a 2 000 lines per mm modulation rate. Therefore in most cases the M T F

of these emulsions is not a limitation.
    * Thickness and index variation of the gelatin :
    They modulate the phase in the reconstructed wave. Mesures (2) have proved that this modulation affects the efficiency of the hologram by a factor of few percents only, for spatial frequencies lower than 1 000 mm^{-1} and even less for spatial frequencies higher than that.
    - linearity :
    In order to accurately reconstruted a wave recorded by holography a linear relation is required between the illumination received by the recording plate and its magnitude transmission.
    This condition is approximated for thin holograms, in a small part of the characteristic curves of this type of emulsion (see characteristic H and D)
    - diffraction efficiency :
    A thin hologram, not bleached, cannot theoretically diffract more than 6,5 % of the incident light.
    For a thin bleached hologram this theoretic number is 34 %.
    For a thick bleached hologram this theoretic number is 100 %.
    However it should be noted that for thickness greater than 50 μm, silver halide emulsions present other problems (sliding and deformation of the gelatin, the difficulty to get the chemical products to penetrate uniformly the gelatin during the processing).
    New emulsions, but above all new chemical processings (U.S.A., England, Netherland) concerning the developer and the bleach yield::
    - stable products in time (without printing),
    - high diffraction efficiencies (> 90 %),
    - high quality images,
    - finally, it should not be forgotten that these emulsions can be laid on very large areas.
    The two main handicaps of this type of materials are that they require a posteriori complex chemical processing and they are not reversible.
    During the last decade emulsions come from KODAK but mainly from AGFA-GEVAERT.
    It should be noted today ILFORD in ENGLAND should market in near futur emulsion especially created for holography, with a better sensitivity in green and in blue and a very good resolution. That is a promising point for the futur of holography.

The dichromated gelatin

    Added with dichromate ammonium (which brings chronium ions C_r^{6+}), the gelatin gets polymerized by the action of the light.
    Because of the low life time of the dichromated gelatin, these materials must be prepared just before use.
    These processes are extremly dependent on external conditions (humidity, temperature, cleanliness...). Many papers give detailed descriptions of preparation used (and the developing procedures are discussed in extend (3), (4),(5), (6).
    In order to conserv holograms in dichromated gelatin it is better to cover them with an adhesive coat of organic resin (7).

Characteristic features of the dichromated gelatin
    - energetic sensitivity :
    It is a very low sensitive material : one thousand times less than silver halide emulsions.
    Special processing lower the quantity of necessary energy to a few tens of J/cm^2. in the blue giving a good diffraction efficiency (about 80 %).
    - spectral sensitivity :
    Near U.V., blue.
    They can be presensibilize with blue of methylen for recording in the green.
    - resolution :
    The dichromated gelatin is an homogenous material, without grain, allowing the recording of at least 6 000 lines/mm.
    - diffration efficiency :
    excellent : > 90 %.
    - response :
    This material remains unequal in terms of diffraction efficiency and signal-to-noise ratio (image contrast).

    Its high resolution makes this material well suited to reflexion holograms.
    The large thickness of the prepared layers makes it suited for multiple storage (H.O.E., filters for phase filtering).
    In spite of all the publications concerning the production, the processing and the conservation of this material, it seems that few teams in the world really tower above all of the procedures (THOMSON CSF, SFENA,... in France ; PILKINGTON,... in England, HUGHES AIRCRAFT,... in U.S.A.,...) which proves the pratical difficulties of their use.

The photoresists

The photoreticulation phenomenum mentioned in connection with the dichromated gelatin may be observed on some other substances, especially resins.

The photoresists are synthetic resins where the restored image, after chemical processing can be formed in two different ways :
- by the regions unexposed to light : positive photoresist,
- by the regions exposed to light : negative photoresist

In the beginning, the photoresists have be developed for photoengraving applications.

General characteristics features

The photoresists are sold in bottle. The user will be responsible for the coating on the substractof his choice and for the processing.

The procedures, that depend of each product, is given by the manufacturer. Commonly :

preparation of the substrat
- ultrasonics cleaning in isopropylic alcool,
- stoving under inert atmosphere (100° - 200° C)

coating of the photoresist
- with a spinner under controled atmosphere
- rotation speed and operation time must be perfectly controled.

anealing
The plate covered with a layer (about 1 µm thick) is heated ($\simeq 100°$C) during 10 to 20 minutes depending of the materials and the processing.

illumination
Near U.V. of far blue

development
- immersion of the plate in a special developer supplied by the manufacturer
- then washing in the water or in a specific bath

fixation
a new anealing ($\simeq 150°$ C) to eliminate the last developer traces and to held the adherence of the photoresist on the substrat.

Characteristics features of the photoresists

energy sensitivity
very low. It is very depending of the wavelength during the exposure (Several J/cm^2 for $\lambda = 448$ nm, few mJ/cm^2 for $\lambda = 355$ nm).

spectral sensitivity
300 to 470 nm

linearity
it is a pur phase material including a phase shift $\Delta \phi (x,y)$:

$$\Delta \phi (x,y) = \frac{2n}{\lambda} (n - 1) \Delta e$$

- r = index of the photoresist
- λ = reading wavelength
- Δe = thikness variation after development

Δe is not a linear function of the illumination, therefore neither is the photoresist

In order to get the good conditions for holography use we must control :
- the thickness of the layer (modulation depth)
- the level of the energetic illumination
- the developer concentration

resolution
can reach 9 000 mm^{-1}

diffraction
the best diffraction efficiency is obtained with a low signal - to - noise ratio. This efficiency is a decreasing function of the resolution.

A good adequation between resolution , signal - to - noise ratio, and diffraction efficiency is : 1 500 mm^{-1}, 20 dB and 10 %.

As a conclusion, the photoresists are low noise and low diffusion materials, which, in the field of phase holography, make them good candidates for the H.O.E. For a small thickness, it is possible to obtain good linearities conditions and therefore are used for the hologram duplication (embossed holograms) and should be used for mass producted H.O.E. in the futur. They allow the realisation of phase profil (kinoforms) for image processing or lens correction or optical system correction.

Their low energetic sensitivity and their spectral sensitivity require long exposure times and the use of U V Sources (Hg lamp and He-Cd laser) or blues sources (Argon laser) with the problem of a lower energetic sensitivity. At this date this two points are a handicap.

They are not reversible.

The main manufacturers are : KODAK, SHIPLEY, GAF.

Concerning the choice of the material, one important critary is the adherence of the photoresist on the substrat, which depends on the product and the type of substrat :
for example : KODAK/KPR : good adherence on copper
                 KODAK/KFTR : good adherence on silicon and on metals
                 SHIPLEY/AZ 1350 : good adherence on aluminium; chromium, S ; 0_2.

The thermoplastics

The use of thermoplastic as recording material for holography was described the first time by URBACH and MEIR.

The proposed technique which has been proved successful, consists in a transparent sandwich : thermoplastic - photoconductor - conductor, used in a mode : load - exposure - reload.

The thermoplastic is coated on a photoconductor and is electrally loaded. Exposed to light which modifies the electrical charge distribution in the neighbourhood of photoconductor, reload and heated nearly at his fusion point. In this way we obtain a relief variation on the thermoplastic surface which geometrically corresponds the field of the recorded fringes.

The general mode operating has now several recording procedures for the different thermoplastic :
- in order to get better diffraction efficiencies
- in order to get more reliable results
- in order to get larger band width.

These results can be combine but influence one an other in a negative way : for exemple a good diffraction efficiency often implies a loss of sensitivity.

Characteristics features of the thermoplastics

energetic sensitivity
more or less as the silver halide materials ($\simeq$ 50 μJ/cm2

spectral sensitivity
easy to sensibilize (doping of the PVK) up to the I.R.

linearity
because of the electrostatic nature of the recording process, there is a band width.
Therefore the thermoplastics behave as a band pass filter.

The position of the peak frequency of the bandwith depends on the thickness of the material and on the magnitude of the electrostatic field: typically from 10 mm^{-1} to 1 000 mm^{-1}

resolution
these materials are generaly used in fixed set ups (i.e. holographic instant camera) and there for optimized with respect to linearity ($\simeq$ 800 mm^{-1})

diffraction efficiency
between 5 % and 30 %, depending on the absorbed quantity of energy by the material.

recyclability
they are erasable and rewritable several thousands times.

More than that a fatigue appears (because the electrical charges deteriorate the material)

The rewritting speed is about a few hundred milliseconds.

As a conclusion, the thermoplastics offer the following avantages :
- they are recyclable several thousands times
- they have a panchromatic sensitivity
- they have a low noise level
- they have a good diffraction efficiency

The holograms obtained with this material are thin phase holograms.

The thermoplastics are well suited for quasi reel time holographic interferometry.

The technical characteristics of the materials are used in two different ways :
- for their recyclability (NEWPORT - RICOH)
- to take advandtage of their dry process (NEWPORT, MICRAUDEL, ROTTENKOWBER)

The photopolymers

They are organic substances generally liquid, in which polymerisation reaction can be exposure to light.

The photopolymers contain three fundamental compounds :
- one monomer able to polymerize
- a photosensitive catalyser
- a catalyser desactivator (same action as photographic fix)

Characteristics features of the photopolymers

energetic sensibility :
good in U.V. : a few mJ/cm^2
decreases in blue : 10 to 20 mJ/cm2

spectral sensitivity :
near U.V. and blue

diffraction efficiency :
The photopolymers allow the recording of thick phase holograms, consequently, theorically, diffraction efficiency : 100 %

Actually, the diffraction efficiency ρ depends on the number of lines per millimeter p, on the illumination energy E, on the thickness of the photopolymer layer e, on the reading wavelength λ_r, on the percentage of activator in the monomer % a :

$$\rho \text{ actual} = f (p, E, e, \lambda_r, \% \frac{a}{m})$$

<u>linearity and resolution</u>

The photopolymers generally exhibit a peek at about 1 500 mm^{-1} and a minima at about 100 mm^{-1}.

The degradable photopolymers

They have the property to be degraded by the action of light.

The main material is the poly methylmethacrylate (PMMA)

The <u>energetic sensitivity</u> is not as good as the above materials but on the other hand they offer a <u>better résolution</u> : several thousands lines per millimeter.

Important efforts have been made for the study and the manufacturing of the materials ; for example, in France by ISSEC, GUILLEMINOT, CNRS,... ; in U.S.A. by HUGHES AIRCRAFT, BELL,...

The main problem encountered until now is its lack of stability, before and after use.

Things seem to be changing since two new photopolymers provide similar results to the dichromated gelatin :
- one of them studied at IBM
- the other has been studied at POLAROID CORPORATION (8),
will be marketed in the near futur. It is refered to under the code DMP - 128. Thin photopolymer can be recorded in the blue (442 nm and 448 nm), in the green (514 nm) and in the red (633 nm and 647 nm).

Its energetic sensibility is very good (5 mJ/cm^2) and diffraction efficiency is between 80 % and 95 %. The refraction index modulation is about 0,03 (which is very good). It should be noted that after the laser exposure an uniform illumination of white light is necessary to terminate the photopolymerisation.

Finally its use is simplified compared to the other photopolymers and offer a good stability in time which removes the majour handicap of the photopolymers.

The photochroms

Under the action of light and heat the photochromic materials change colour in a reversible manner. This faculty can be taken advantage to use as a recording material.

The operating procedure is then :

$\lambda_1 \rightarrow$ writing
$\lambda_2 \rightarrow$ reading
$\lambda_3 \rightarrow$ erasing

They are two types of photochroms : the organic photochromic material (spirospyran, mercury dithizomate, anil) and the non organic photochromic materials (sulphus,)

Their <u>energetic sensitivity</u> is low (0,1 J/cm^2 at λ = 500 nm) because there is no "developer" therefore there is no amplification.

Their <u>resolution</u> is very good, because the size of the molecules are much smaller that the size of the diffraction spot.

However numerous problems remain :
- during the reading a progressive destruction of the stored information occurs
- the life time of the excited state is limited , even at an ambiant temperature (from several seconds to several days)
- the aptitude of the photochrom to pass from a state to an other decreases as the inverse of the number of cycles undergone by the material.

The fatigue effect is the main limit for the use of the photochroms.

The electro-optical crystals

As far as the study of erasable and reversible materials for the optical storage of information is concerned , two types of applications are considered :
- the binary storage of information on a disc
- image recording on or in medium allowing a fast processing of information.

In this paper we will only be concerned with the second case, and in this case we will only investigate the optical processing of optical information using holography. That is a field which has been and which becomes again intensitivity studied. One simplified set up is presented figure 1.

This processing set up, theoritically very efficient (high speed and high capability: parallel architecture and photons) has always been penalized by :
1 - the data imput (incoherent - coherent)
2 - the difficulty to dispose of a quasi real time holographic recording material, to be introduce in the filter plane (Fourier plane).

The solution of point 1 can be opproached as an example with the optical valve.

In order to attempt solving point 2, the photorefractive materials offer extensively exploited (9).

The photorefractive materials are crystalline materials able to become birefringent under the action of an electrical field.

This capability is exploited to record a luminous phenomenum. (the some process is used in there modulators.

The main crystals which present the best photorefractive qualities are :

$Li Nb O_3$ <u>Energetic sensibility</u>
low $\simeq 10 J/cm^2$

$La Ti O_3$ better if doping with $Fe_2O_3 \simeq 1$ to 3 J/cm^2
refer to Thomson CSF which is the company the most involved in the world : especially to use them to create a RAM

$Bi_{12} Si O_{20}$ (BSO)   <u>energetic sensitivity</u>

$Bi_{12} Ge O_{20}$ (BGO)   more better than $Li No O_3$ $\simeq 150$ $\mu J/cm^2$
in general $\simeq 300$ $\mu/J cm^2$

$Ba Ti O_3$ <u>high resolution</u> $\simeq 1\ 000$ mm^{-1}

But there is a life time problem
This material find their applications in holography interferometry, metrology logy, image processing (12) (13) (14).

S B N   refer to works of Taxter and Micheron (15) (16)
K T N

PLZT   They are ceramics ; their main advantage is the fact that can be manufacture with larger dimensions than the monocrystal.

CdS

     <u>spectral sensitivity</u>
Blue and green for the doped crystals with Fe^{2+} , red for those doped with Co
<u>storage capacity</u>
theoritically : 10^8 bits/cm^2 - 10^{12} bits/cm^3.
actually : 10^7 bits/cm^2 - 10^{10} bits/cm^3.
which corresponds, by mean of the thick holograms property, to be able theoritically several hundred holograms in one cubic centimeter, but actually, the fact that these crystals are erasable under the action of the intense light field (fifteen times more intense that during writing) limits this value.

<u>diffration efficiency</u>
it is theoritically high but actually limited in the applications for which the electro-optical crystals are most often used (high number of holograms recorded in the same crystal).

This efficiency is 1 % for about 100 holograms.
<u>writing and erasing time</u>
20 milliseconds for each
<u>recyclability</u>
infinite
no fatigue is observed in the material
<u>linearity</u>
the transfer function can be modify to varying the electrical field applied to the crystal.

Problems:
     - the reading with the same wave length as for the writing tends to erase the hologram
     - the reading with different wavelength than for writing introduces abberations (this is related with Bragg's conditions).
     - the energetic sensitivity remains low in most crystals.
     - the manufacturing of homognous crystal remains difficult
     - the crystallin structure of the photorefractive materials does not allow, generally, to use them on large areas for image recording .

Futur possibilities:
     - a new possibility comes the superlattices which present photorefractive properties. Their evaluation requires a better understanding of the physical phenomene bivolded.
     - the use of space technology, in connections with microgravity (refer to the experiments made aboard the space shuttle open perhaps other new possibilities.

The metallic film

Several of this materials are listed here for memory
     - thin tellurium films   Philips Lab/U.S.A.

- samarium monosulphide films
- vanadium oxide films
- Eu O films } U R S S
- SmS thin films
- Mn Bi films   U R S S + West Germany

It does not seem at this time that either one may be developed for the holographic applications

Conclusion

The silver halid and dichromated gelatins are still extensively used in many applications.

The photoresists technics have reached a mature state which makes them operational

The new photopolymers are interesting for the recording of the volum holograms without grain.

Of course the crystalline medium in which the résults are obtained just after the recording exhibit a sustained interest for the futur of holography. Research programs, for materials to come, are required if one wants that the components of optical processing of the information become reliable and become a basic part of a computer.

We writed in the introduction that the research on new materials is depending on the estimated futur success of such and such application of holography. It is important to point out the event of mass produced holograms. This facts may modify the perception and the impact of the holography, in two supposed ways :

- to supply an image or to diffract front (classical holography)
- or to create new holographic elements generated by the recording of holograms whose form would be modify, by chemical processing during the mastering, or during the embossing.

References

(1) : K. BIEDERMAN - Topics in Applied Physics, 20, H.M. SMITH Editor
        Springer, Berlin, 1977
(2) : H.T.BUCKMANN - Photo Science and Engineering, 13, 425, 1972
(3) : R.G. BRANDES, E.E. FRANCOIS, T.A.S. TANKOFF. Appl. Opt., 8, 2346, 1969
(4) : A. ALFERNESS, S.K. CASE, J. Opt. Soc. Amer., 65, 730, 1975
(5) : D. MEYERHOFER, R.C.A. Review, 33, 110, 1972
(6) : B.J. CHANG, Opt. Commun., 17, 270, 1976
(7) : D.G. Mc CAULEY, C.E. SIMPSON, W.J. MURBACH, App. Opt. 12, 232, 1973
(8) : R.T. INGWALL, H.L. FIELDING, SPIE Vol. 523, p. 306 - 1985
(9) : Final Report, Contrat n° 19 - 73 - C - 0273, Naval Air Systems R.C.A.
(10): PATTERSON and al., Appl. Phys. Letters, 19, 130, 1972
(11): J.P. HUIGNARD, J.P. HERRIAU, F. MICHERON, Appl. Phys. Letters, 26, 5, 1975
(12): H.J. TIZIANI, Optica Acta, 29, 4, 463 - 470, 1982
(13): J.P. HUIGNARD, J.P. HERRIAU, L. PICHON, A. MARRACHI, Opt. Letters, 5, 10, 1980
(14): J.P. HUIGNARD, A. MARRACHI, Opt. Letters, 6, 12, 1981
(15): T.B. TAXTER, M. KESTIGAN, Appl. Opt. 13, 913, 1974
(16): MICHERON and al., Appl. Phys. Letters, 26, 5, 1975

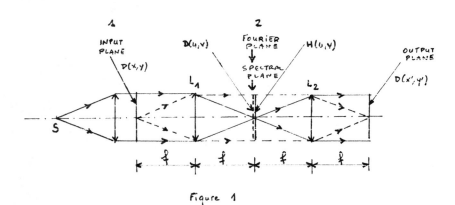

Figure 1

Holographic optical elements using polyvinyl carbazole holographic material

K. Matsumoto, T. Kuwayama, *M. Matsumoto and N. Taniguchi

Canon Research Center, Canon Inc.
5, Morinosato-Wakamiya, Atsugishi, Kanagawa 243-01, Japan
*Reprographic Products Group, Canon Inc.
3-30-2, Shimomaruko, Ohta-ku, Tokyo 146, Japan

Abstract

We developed a new holographic material: polyvinyl carbazole material. The advantage of the material over conventional DCG material is that it has high durability against humidity and transparency. Some optical properties of the material and some applications are presented. We have already installed the holographic display element using polyvinyl carbazole in a commercialized 8mm movie camera. The letters "END" are displayed on an imaging plane of the finder system by using an image plane hologram. We also present the holographic lens of which aberration is well corrected at laser diode wavelength. We made this holographic lens using a new aberration correcting method.

Introduction

The holographic optical elements (HOE) are useful because of their thin film structure, easiness for integration with other optical elements, and mass productivity. The HOE has already been applied to the scanner[1], the coupler of optical fiber[2] and the display element[3]. Furthermore, holographic lenses are expected to be used as a pick-up lens for optical memory unit. The recording materials of the HOE are usually silver halide emulsions, dichromated gelatin films and photopolymer, etc. Among these materials, dichromated gelatin is widely used because of its high diffraction efficiency. However, the drawback of the material is low sensitivity and low durability against humidity. We developed a new holographic recording material mainly consisting of polyvinyl carbazole (PVCz). The new PVCz holographic material is useful because of the high diffraction efficiency and the high durability against humidity.

We applied to one product: 8mm movie camera wich installs the HOE called Superimposed Finder Display (SFD) since 1979. We are now researching the holographic pick-up lens of an optical head.

In this paper, we present the optical properties of the PVCz holographic recording material. The SFD[4] and the holographic lens[5] with the PVCz holographic material are also shown.

PVCz holographic recording material

We show the process chart for obtaining the HOE of the PVCz material in Fig.1. PVCz is sensitized by using carbon tetraiodide. Carbon tetraiodide is incorporated in PVCz and constitutes the sensitive material having a sufficient sensitivity in a visible wavelength region. The sensitized PVCz material is coated on the glass plate with a spinner in the dark room. The thickness of the coated film is about $6\mu m$ after drying. The holographic plate is exposed by an Ar ion laser (wavelength 488nm). Carbon tetraiodide generates radicals when the sensitive material is exposed. According to the intensity distribution of the incident light, the radicals cause a crosslinking reaction between the polymers. The crosslinking causes the difference of the degree of polymerization. Then the interference pattern is transferred to the pattern of crosslinking.

The holographic plate is developed by two kind of solvent treatment. The sensitive material is swelled by the first solvent. The sensitizer is removed from the material at the same time. The second solvent treatment causes the shrinking of the swelled sensitive material. In this manner, the high diffraction efficiency phase hologram is obtained. Then it is covered with a glass plate for protecting the PVCz film.

Preparation of holographic material
↓ (PVCz + Carbon tetraiodide)
Coating with spinner
↓
Exposure
↓ (Ar ion laser wavelength 488nm)
Development
↓ (Solvent treatment)
Covering with a glass plate

Fig.1 The procedure of producing the H.O.E using the PVCz material

Characteristics of the PVCz holographic recording material

The spectral sensitivity of the photosensitive material is shown in Fig.2. It was measured by employing Grating Spectrograph, RM-23-1 (manufactured by NALUMI Co. Ltd.). The longest limit of recordable wavelength is 560 nm.

The diffraction efficiency of the hologram vs. the exposed energy is shown in Fig.3. The sensitivity at 488 nm of an Ar ion laser is excellent. The practically satisfactory diffraction efficiency of 35 % is obtained only by 10 mJ/cm^2 of exposure energy. The maximum diffraction efficiency (96 %) is obtained by the exposure of 50 mJ/cm^2. The exposure exceeding 50 mJ/cm^2 diminishes the diffraction efficiency of holograms.

The durability test of the PVCz hologram which has no protecting glass plate is done in high humidity and temperature atmosphere; 70°C 95% R.H. The change of the diffraction efficiency vs. the time elapsed is shown in Fig.4. Even after the elapse of one month (720 hours), the diffraction efficiency of the hologram is little diminished. As the commercialized HOE is covered with the protecting glass plate, then the durability characteristics are improved more than the naked hologram.

Fig.5 shows the spectroscopic transmittance of the PVCz hologram. Transmittance of 91 % is obtained at the wavelength of He-Ne laser (632.8 nm). This transmittance shows how this material is clear in visible spectrum.

In addition, the resolution (3500 lines/mm) of the PVCz holographic material is superior to those of the other materials. The drawback of this material is that shelf life is very short. The sensitivity of this material is diminished day by day and the limitation of use is 7 days.

Above mentioned characteristics of this material are summarized in Table 1.

Subject	Characteristics	Condition
Recording wavelength range	< 560 nm	
Sensitivity	10 mJ/cm^2	at wavelength 488 nm diffraction efficiency = 35 %
Maximum diffraction efficiency	97 % 89 %	at wavelength 633 nm at wavelength 820 nm Thickness of sensitive material = 6 μm
Transmittance	91 % 93 %	at wavelength 633 nm at wavelength 820 nm
Resolution	> 3500 lines/mm	
Durability against temperature and humidity	Unchanged	70°C 95% R.H. 720 hours without protecting glass plate

Table 1. Characteristics of the PVCz holographic recording material

Holographic optical elements (HOE) using the PVCz holographic material

Superimposed information display in a commercialized 8mm movie camera

We developed a new finder system with the HOE, called SFD (Superimposed Finder Display), using the PVCz holographic material. The new holographic element SFD which can display the letters "END" in an imaging plane of the finder system has already been installed in a commercialized 8mm movie camera (Canon 1014XL-S) since 1979. The letters "END" are displayed by illuminating the hologram with a tungsten lamp. Under normal conditions of the camera, the tungsten lamp is turned off, then the letters "END" are invisible, and one can continue shooting. When the film ends, the letters "END" are displayed in the viewfinder. These letters "END" become clearly visible in the viewfinder, overlapping the image field, giving a colorful and amazing warning emerged by the PVCz hologram.

Fig.6 shows the viewfinder displaying the letters "END". This function is not possible to be realized by conventional display elements, such as LED and liquid crystal.

Fig.7 shows optical system which contains the HOE for SFD. The hologram is placed in the image plane of the finder system. The hologram is illuminated by a tungsten lamp. The light is diffracted at the portion of letters "END" which has grating structure and comes into the eyepiece. Then it is possible to observe the letters "END" as a colored bright image through the eyepiece. Necessarily, the light from an imaging lens to form finder image is also diffracted by the hologram. If the diffraction efficiency of the hologram is high, the letters "END" are observed as a "shadow". This problem can be prevented by diminishing the diffraction efficiency and utilizing the shallow angular selectivity of the Bragg hologram.

This hologram is produced by the step and repeat method which is suitable for mass

production. The holographic plate (3x3 inches) is exposed by an Ar ion laser light, and the letters "END" of 25 pieces are recorded in some 3 minutes.
Fig.8 shows the sample of the hologram in which the letters "END" of 25 pieces are recorded.

Off-axis holographic lens for a laser diode

It is especially desirable that the HOE is able to be used at the wavelength of laser diode. However, we do not have suitable holographic material which has sensitivity at the wavelength of a laser diode (nearly 800 nm). When the holographic lens is made by the light from a short wavelength laser and used at long wavelength, large aberration appears due to the difference between recording and reconstructing wavelengths. We develcped a method of correcting the aberration of an off-axis holographic lens, as well as an in-line holographic lens[7], which is caused by the wavelength difference. This method is accomplished by introducing a predetermined aberration into the object wave when the holographic lens is made. The predetermined aberration of an off-axis holographic lens is generated by a plane-parallel glass plate placed in converging beam of hologram-making arrangement shown in Fig.9.
The converging wave (object wave) with the desired aberration is obtained by a photographic objective 50 mm f/1.2 and a plane-parallel glass plate of 27.7 mm thickness. The PVCz holographic material is illuminated by an Ar ion laser light of 488 nm. The focal length of the holographic lens is 3.5 mm and a value of N.A. is 0.48.
Fig.10 shows the measured profile of the intensity distribution of a light spot at the focal plane of the holographic lens reconstructed with a laser diode (wavelength is 820 nm). The $1/e^2$ diameter of the measured light spot is 1.8 μm and 30 % greater than the theoretical value. The diffraction efficiency of the lens is about 8 %. The diffraction efficiency of the lens will be able to be increased over 80 % using the Bragg-angle shift copy method.

Conclusion

We developed a polyvinyl carbazole (PVCz) holographic recording material. The optical properties of the PVCz material is superior to those of the other materials because of high diffraction efficiency, high durability against humidity and temperature, high resolution and mass productivity of the PVCz holograms.
Mass production of the holographic elements was realized by the step and repeat printing method and due to the advantage of the PVCz holographic material. The holographic optical element called Superimposed Finder Display has already been installed in a commercialized 8mm movie camera.
We obtained the aberration corrected off-axis holographic lens that has a near diffraction-limited spot at the laser diode wavelength. The holographic lens will be put to practical use in the near future.

Acknowledgements

The authors wish to express their sincere thanks to Katsuhiko Nishide, Takashi Tanaka, Koujiro Yokono, Shigeo Toganou and Hiroyoshi Kishi for the development of the new holographic material, and also to Sachiko Igarashi for helping our experiments. The authors also wish to thank Kiyonobu Endo for his helpful discussion and encouragement.

References

1. I. Cindrich : Appl. Opt. 6, 153 (1967).
2. H. Nishihara, S. Inohara, T.Suhara, and J. Koyama : IEEE J. Quant. Electron. QE-11, 9, 794 (1975).
3. D. Meyerhofer : Appl. Opt. 12, 2180 (1973).
4. K. Matsumoto and S. Matsumura : SPIE 193, 198 (1979).
5. T. Kuwayama, Y. Nakamura, N. Taniguchi, and S. Suda : ICO-13 C6-6 (1984).
6. U.S. Patent, No.4172724
7. G. N. Buinov and K. S. Mustafin : Opt. Spectrosc. 41,90 (1976).

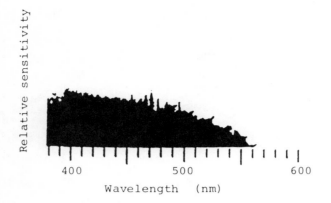

Fig.2 The spectral sensitivity of the PVCz
holographic recording material

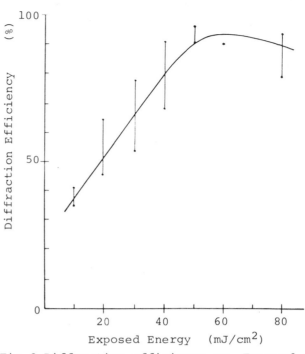

Fig.3 Diffraction efficiency vs. Exposed energy
of the PVCz holographic material

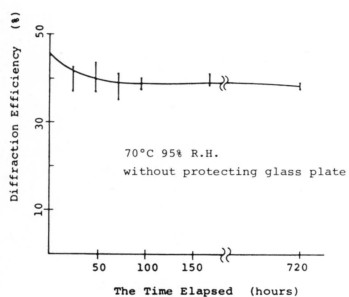

70°C 95% R.H.

without protecting glass plate

Fig.4 The result of durability test against
temperature and humidity of the PVCz
hologram

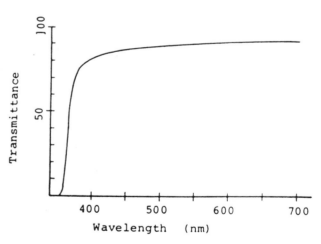

Fig.5 The spectroscopic transmittance of
the PVCz hologram

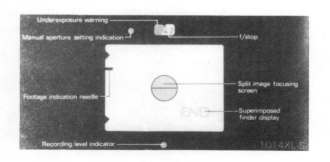

Fig.6 The viewfinder displaying the letters "END"
in a commercialized 8mm movie camera

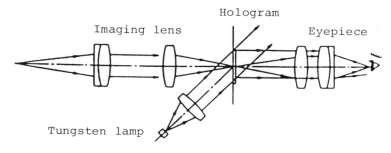

Fig.7 Superimposed Finder Display System
with a hologram

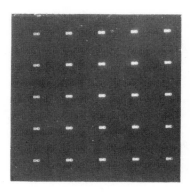

Fig.8 The PVCz hologram produced
by the step and repeat method

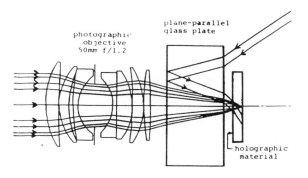

Fig.9 The optical system for recording
the holographic lens

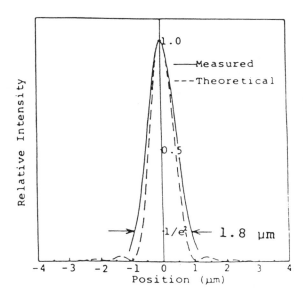

Fig.10 Relative intensity distribution of
a spot reconstructed with a holographic
lens

Holographic recording material containing poly-N-vinylcarbazole

Yasuo Yamagishi, Takeshi Ishizuka, Teruo Yagishita,
Kasumi Ikegami, and Hirofumi Okuyama

FUJITSU LABORATORIES LTD.
Morinosato Wakamiya, Atsugi 243-01, Japan

Abstract

A volume phase holographic recording material with high diffraction efficiency and high durability against humidity has been developed.

The holographic material consists of Poly-N-vinylcarbazole (PVCz) as a base polymer, camphorquinone as an initiator and thioflavine-T as a sensitizer.

This film is sensitive to argon ion laser light, and exposure energy of 500 mJ/cm^2 is required to realize high diffraction efficiency. After recording a latent image of a fringe pattern by exposure, a hologram was developed by swelling and shrinking of the film with two sorts of solvent.

The thickness of the hologram could be reduced to 2.5 μm, because the PVCz hologram has a large amplitude of the refractive index modulation related with the crystallinity modulation. The high diffraction efficiency coupled with the thin layer made an incident light angle wide enough to maintain a high diffraction efficiency around the Bragg angle.

Introduction

Silver halide emulsions[1,2] and dichromated gelation[3] are well known as high diffraction efficiency holographic recording materials, for all directions of incident polarized light. These materials require a relatively thick film, thickerthan 6 μm, to obtain high diffraction efficiency of more than 70%, because of small refractive index modulation. However a thick volume phase hologram reduces diffraction efficiency when the incident light angle of the reconstructed light shifts slightly from the Bragg angle. This reduction of the diffraction efficiency restricts use for various applications of a holography. Moreover those materials which are made of water soluble gelatin, have poor humidity resistance. A hologram made of these materials will need a tough cover against humidity.

The purpose of our work was to develop a new holographic recording material with high diffraction efficiency using thin holographic film and with high humidity resistance.

We chose Poly-N-vinylcarbazole (PVCz) as a polymer for the holographic material because of its high refractive index and its high durability against humidity. We studied sensitization and fabricating method of the PVCz hologram. In this paper we discuss holographic properties, refractive index modulation, and durability against humidity of the PVCz hologram.

Experimental

Materials

Commercially available Poly-N-vinylcarbazole (Tuvicol 210, Anan Kouryo LTD.) and camphorquinone (Eastman Kodak) were used in this study without purification. Thioflavine-T (Kanto Chmical Co.Inc.), used as a sensitizer, was purified by recrystallization, using ethylalcohol. A certain amount of PVCz, camphorquinone, and thioflavinn-T were dissolved in a good solvent, then filtered with a 3 μm pore filter. The composition of the solution is shown in Table 1. Photosensitive PVCz film was spin-coated from the solution to a thickness of 1.4 μm and dried in a nitrogen atmosphere at room temperature.

Fabricating method

Latent holographic patterns were recorded into the photosensitive PVCz film using the exposing system shown in Figure 1. In this system, an Ar laser beam (λ=488 nm) was devided into two beams with equivalent energy. Then the beams were expanded and collimated to 5 cm diameter. Using the mirrors, an adequate spatial frequency was adjusted to make the required diffraction gratings. The exposure intensity on the film was about 6 mw/cm^2.

After exposure, the film was developed by the following process (Figure 2).
(1) Pretreatment: Almost all the camphorquinone and thioflavine-T in the film was extracted with ethylalcohol.
(2) Swelling: The PVCz film was swelled by the good solvent (toluen) for PVCz.
(3) Shrinking: After swelling, the swelled PVCz film was dipped into the poor solvent (pentane).

Measurements

Diffraction efficiency for a He-Ne Lesar beam was measured with a silicon photo-diode as the detector. The incident light angle to the holographic film was set so as to maximize the first-order diffraction intensity.

As one of photochemical properties of the sensitized PVCz film, the light absorption spectrum was measured with a spectrophotometer.

To study the recording mechanism of the volume phase hologram, crystallinity and reffractive index differences of the film before and after exposure were examined. Crystallinity was evaluated by the difference in X-ray diffraction patterns. Reffractive index was estimated from the shift in the interferrometric fringe photographed with an interferrometric microscope.

Durability of the hologram was evaluated from the diffraction efficiency change under environmental conditions of 40°C and 95% R.H.

Results and discussion

Holographic properties of the PVCz hologram

Figure 3 shows a typical absorption spectrum of 1.4 µm thick sensitized and nonsensitized PVCz films. From Figure 3, it was found that thioflavine-T enabled the PVCz hologram to absorb argon ion laser light.

Figure 4 shows exposure energy dependence on diffraction efficiency. From Figure 4, an exposure energy of about 500 mJ/cm^2 is required to obtain the highest diffraction efficiency. The PVCz hologram has a first-order diffraction efficiency (η) of 80%, and has less than 5% zeroth-order diffraction efficiency. Incident light of 12% is reflected by the surface of the substrate.

The diffraction efficiency is also strongly affected by the spatial frequency of the holographic grating. Figure 5 shows that relationship between η and spatial frequency. η of more than 60% is retained between 800 2500 line/mm. This high diffraction efficiency suggests that a volume phase hologram is formed in PVCz film.

Figure 6 shows the relationship between η and the incident angle of the He-Ne laser beam. The highest diffraction efficiency is obtained when the incident angle is the Bragg angle. With an increase of the shift of incident angle from the Bragg angle, the η decreases. $\Delta\theta$ in Figure 6 is the half bandwidth of the η. $\Delta\theta$ is related to fringe spacing, d, and hologram thickness, t, as follows[4],

$$\Delta\theta \simeq d/t \qquad (1)$$

According to the equation (1), $\Delta\theta$ decreases as hologram thickness increases for the same fringe spacing. Owing to the thin film, 2.5 µm, $\Delta\theta$ of the PVCz hologram shown in Figure 6 is larger than that of bleached silver halide holographic film.

So the PVCz hologram can maintain high diffraction efficiency. It is thought that the PVCz hologram will be applied for optical elements, even when the incident angle must shift from the Bragg angle due to the device design.

Refractive index modulation of the PVCz film

To clarify the reason why thin PVCz hologram has a high diffraction efficiency, we measured the refractive index of exposed and unexposed areas after development. Peeling a part of the PVCz film formed on silicon wafer, we observed the PVCz film and the peeled part of the wafer at the same time with an interferrometric micrometer. Figure 7 shows the inter-ferrometric fringes of the exposed and unexposed areas. In each photograph, the left part is the PVCz film and the right part is the substrate. A and B in Figure 7 indicate the shifted number of the fringe due to phase shift. We obtained 1.50 as the refractive index in the unexposed area. In the same way, we obtained 1.82 as the refractive index in the region exposed to a single Ar laser beam. From these results, we obtained 0.32 as the index difference between exposed and unexposed areas. This index difference indicates the maximum index modulation of the PVCz hologram. However this index difference does not indicate the index modulation of the actual hologram. To determine the quantity of the index modulation in an actual hologram, we tried to determine the index modulation (Δn) from the diffraction efficiency of the PVCz film. Theoretical diffraction efficiency expected from a certain thickness of the hologram can be calculated from a following relation,

$$\eta' = \frac{I_1}{I_0} \times 100$$
$$= \sin^2\left(\frac{\pi (\Delta n/2)^2 t}{\lambda \cos\theta}\right) \qquad (2)$$

where Δn is the amplitude of the index modulation, t is the hologram thickness, and θ indicates the angle between object and reference beams.

In equation (2), 2.5 μm, 1 (a low angle), 438 nm, and 88% are substituted for t, cos θ, λ, and η' repectively and Δn = 0.24 is obtained.

In order to know the reason for this large Δn, we observed the X-ray diffraction curves shown in Figure 8. A crystalline diffraction peak at $2\theta = 40.2°$ appeared in the developed film. The peak value of the exposed area of the developed film was higher than that of the unexposed area of the developed film. This fact shows that the index modulation is formed by the crystallinity of the PVCz film. Also, from the peak angle, it was found that the spacing of the PVCz crystal structure was 2.8 Å, because λ = 1.937 Å and θ = 20.1° for 2 d sin θ = nλ. This result suggests that the large index modulation of the PVCz hologram is generated by a modulation of the crystallinity of the PVCz.

Figure 9 shows a cross section of a hologram film. This photograph was taken by illuminating the PVCz hologram from behind. It is obvious from Figure 9 that a volume phase hologram was formed in the PVCz film. The grating-like structure shows the modualtion of the refractive index in the PVCz layer.

Durability against humidity

Figure 10 shows the humidity resistance. Several PVCz holograms with no covers were exposed to 40°C and 95% R.H. As shown in Figure 10, a high diffraction efficiency was kept for more than 1000 hours. The PVCz holograms will be applied as optical elements without any covers against humidity.

Conclusion

A new recording material for volume phase holograms has been developed. PVCz was selected as the base polymer because of its high refractive index and its high durability against humidity. The medium also consisted of camphorquinone as an initiator and thioflavine-T as a sensitizer. The medium is sensitive to argon ion lasers (λ = 488 nm), and the required exposure energy for η of 80% is 500 mJ/cm^2.

A feature of the PVCz hologram is very high diffraction efficiency of 70% at the spatial frequencies of 1000 ∿ 2000 line/mm. The thickness of the hologram can be reduced to 2.5 μm, because the difference of the refractive index between exposed and unexposed areas is larger than 0.3 after development. So the PVCz hologram has wide torelance of incident light angle around the Bragg angle.

The other topical feature of the PVCz hologram is high durability against humidity. High diffraction efficiency was kept for more than 1000 hours, under 40°C and 95% R.H. The PVCz hologram will be applied for various kinds of holographic optical elements.

Aknowledgements

The authors would like to thank Dr. Z. Henmi, Dr. T. Inagaki, Dr. F. Yamagishi, Mr. H. Ikeda and Mr. T. Narusawa for their discussion and encouragement during the course of this work. Thanks are also due to Mr. A. Mochizuki for his support in this work.

References

1. Juris Upatnieks and Carl Leonard, "Diffraction Efficiency of Bleached Photographically Recorded Intereference Patterns", Appl. Opt. Vol. 8 No. 1 pp.85-89 1969

2. A. Graube, "Advances in Bleaching Methods for Photographically Recorded Holograms", Appl. Opt. Vol. 13 No. 12 pp.2942-2946 1974

3. S. K. Case and R. Alferness., "Index Moduration and Spatial Harmonic Generation on Dicromated Geratin Films," Appl. Phys., Vol. 40, pp.41-51. 1976

4. H. Kogelnik., "Coupled Wave Theory for Thick Hologram Grating," Bell.Sys.Tech.J., Vol. 48, pp.2909-2947. 1969

Table 1   The composition of photosensitive solutions

	Material	Content (g)
Matrix polymer	PVCz	100
Reactive initiator	Camphorquinone	24
Sensitizer	Thioflavine-T	3
Solvent	Chloroform	2500

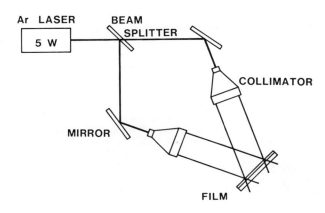

Figure 1   The exposure system for the PVCz hologram

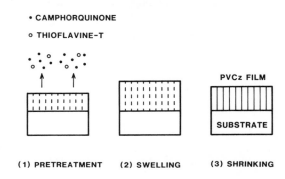

Figure 2   Developing process of the PVCz hologram

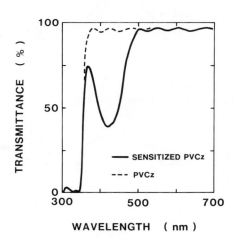

Figure 3   Absorption spectrum of the PVCz film

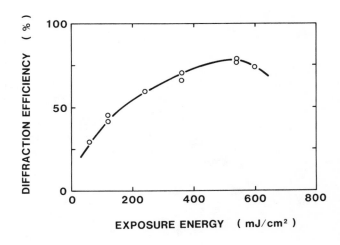

Figure 4   Exposure energy dependence on the diffraction efficiency

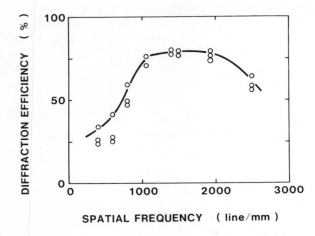

Figure 5   Spatial frequency dependence
on the diffraction
efficiency

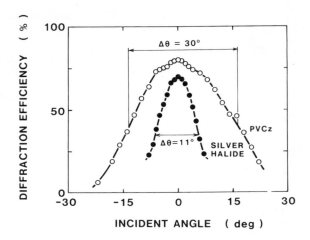

Figure 6   The relationship between
incident angle and
diffraction efficiency
The PVCz hologram has higher diffraction
efficiency than bleached silver
halide for wide shift angle around
the Bragg angle.

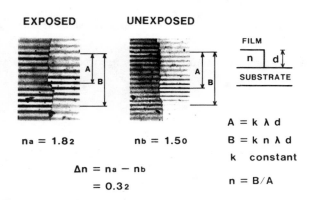

$n_a = 1.8_2$ $n_b = 1.5_0$

$A = k \lambda d$

$B = k n \lambda d$

k constant

$\Delta n = n_a - n_b$

$= 0.3_2$

$n = B/A$

Figure 7   The refractive index difference between exposed and unexposed films.
The PVCz film was developed after exposure to a single beam.

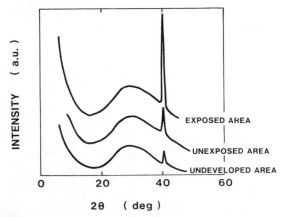

Figure 8   X-ray diffraction spectra of the PVCz hologram
The top is the spectrum of the developed area with exposure.
The middle is the spectrum of the developed area without exposure.
The bottom is the spectrum of the undeveloped area.

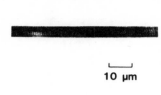

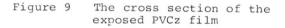

CROSS SECTION

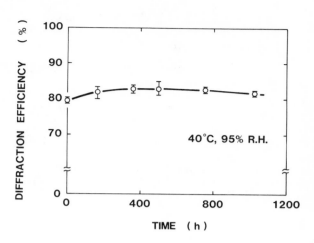

Figure 9   The cross section of the exposed PVCz film

Figure 10   The durability against humidity of the PVCz hologram

Photoelectrochemical etching of holographic gratings in semiconductors and applications

J. Ph. Schnell, V. Martin, P. Nyeki, B Loiseaux, G. Illiaquer, J.P. Huignard

Thomson-CSF, Laboratoire Central de Recherches
Domaine de Corbeville, B.P. n° 10   91401 Orsay Cedex (France)

Abstract

We describe and analyse the use of the photoelectrochemical etching technique to create holographic relief gratings and patterns in semiconductors such as GaAs. Images and wavefront diffracted in the visible and the I.R. will be shown.

Introduction

Laser electrochemical etching of semiconductors raises an increasing interest for the design of high speed electronics and optoelectronic devices. Several applications were mentionned in a recent past : via-holes drilling for microwave integrated circuits[1], InP mesas for millimeter waves transferred electron oscillators[2], etching of integral lenses for diode lasers[3], etching of diffraction gratings for D.F.B. lasers[4], etc.

The basic process is the dissolution of the semiconductor (GaAs, InP, Si...) in a solution (often an oxydizing acidic solution) controlled by the photogenerated carriers under illumination at energies higher than the bandgap. Etching rates of the order of 1 μm/min are obtainable in GaAs, for example, with a moderate illumination (250 mW/cm^2) in the visible. By spatially modulating the light intensity, one can induce a modulation of the etching rate resulting in a relief engraved in the semiconductor. Optical recording of interference or mask projection patterns, in the visible range, is thus possible.

The photoelectrochemical etching of semiconductors is well adapted to realize optical diffractive elements working in the visible and in the infrared, which require several microns size reliefs.

The interest of such deep relief gratings working with wavelength of the same order of magnitude as the spacing is to show high diffraction efficiencies as predicted by the electromagnetic theory[5]. The diffracted energy can be concentrated on one or few orders with an efficiency up to 90 %.

Interesting applications exist such as off-axis optical elements (e.g. : beam multiplexer) and thin holographic lenses.

In this paper, we describe the photoelectrochemical etching in n-GaAs of elementary relief gratings with spacing and depth chosen to optimize the first order diffraction efficiency at 10.6 μm. Their infrared optical characterization is then presented, as well as holographic image recording and readout in the visible.

Photoelectrochemical etching of gratings

The grating etching was realized by projecting an interference fringes pattern onto a (100) oriented n-doped GaAs wafer (dopant : Si ; n=2 to 4×10^{18} cm^{-3}). Fringes were parallel to the [0$\bar{1}$1] axis contained in this plane. The crystal was immersed in a H_2SO_4 : H_2O_2 : H_2O solution with composition 1 : 1 : 100, at room temperature (25 °C).

Interference fringes are produced by the optical set-up shown on the figure 1. The blue line ($\lambda = 488$ nm) of a 2 W - Ar$^+$ laser is used. The laser beam is splitted in two beams which are then expanded and interfere on the sample. The fringe spacing Λ determined by the angle θ between the two beams by $\Lambda = \lambda / 2\sin\theta$, was $\Lambda = 9.5$ μm.

The spatial variation of the intensity is given by $I = I_0 (1 + \cos 2\pi x/\Lambda)$ where I_0 is the total intensity. I_0 was adjusted to 250 mW/cm^2.

Various gratings were created with etching times from 1 to 8 min . The depth is proportionnal to the etching time giving a rate of about 0.75 μm/min . This corresponds to a quantum yield of 26 % (Each GaAs molecule dissolution requires 6 photons). A 100 % quantum yield would correspond to a 10 J/cm^2 writing energy for 1 μm depth.

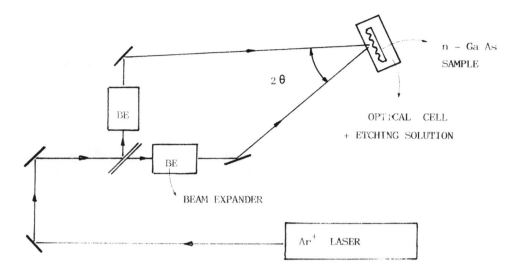

Figure 1. Optical set-up for the photoelectrochemical etching of gratings

On the figure 2 is presented the SEM micrograph of the cross section of a 5 min – etched grating. The created relief, with an amplitude of 3.8 μm, shows roughly the same sinusoïdal profile as the light intensity.

Profiles and etch rates are sensitive to the relative orientation of the fringes and the $[0\bar{1}1]$ cristallographic axis : a 90° rotation was observed to lower the etch rate by 50 % giving sharper gratings.

The etching time can be lowered by raising the temperature : at 45 °C the etch rate is increased by 65 % ; this suggests some rate limitation by the interfacial reaction or the reactants transport. By optimizing the solution composition (with three times larger H_2O_2 concentration), increased etch rate (1.4 μm/min) are obtained. The profile becomes also more triangular.

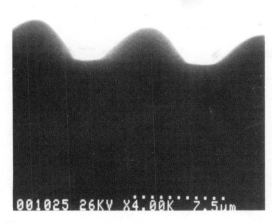

Figure 2. SEM micrograph of a photo-etched grating in n- GaAs (cross section)

I.R. Characterization

Once metallized, the photo-etched gratings were characterized at $\lambda = 10.6$ μm. The optical set-up is described in the figure 3 : a 4W - CO_2 laser creates a beam the intensity and the polarization of which can be adjusted by two half-wavelength plates and a plate under Brewster incidence. The grating is fixed on a rotating holder allowing the incidence angle to be varied. The diffracted and reflected intensities are measured on a pyrodetector.

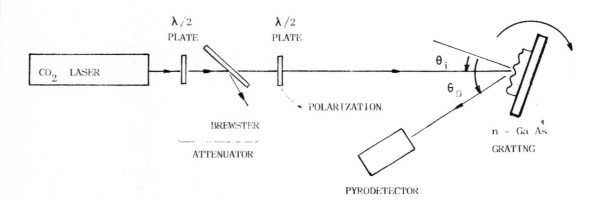

Figue 3. Optical set-up for infrared characterization of gratings

The figure 4 shows the measured zero and 1st order efficiency variations as a function of the incidence angle (from 15° to 45°) corresponding to a grating with 9.5 μm spacing, 4.5 μm depth and a roughly sinusoïdal profile (etching with fringes parallel to the [0Ī1] cristallographic axis).

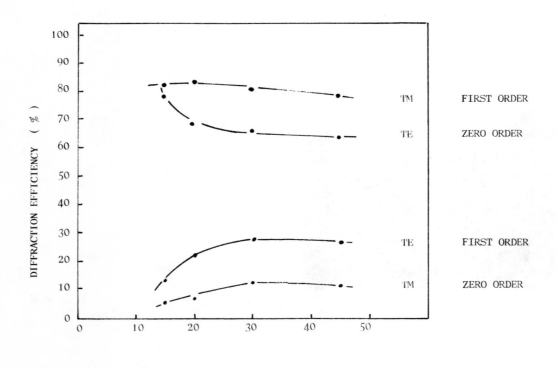

Figure 4. 0 and 1st order diffraction efficiencies of a roughly sinusoïdal grating (spacing : 9.5 μm ; depth : 4.5 μm) at $\lambda = 10.6$ μm.

The measured first order efficiency in TM mode are higher than 80% ou the whole explored incidence angles range. These high values are close to the theoretical ones. The zero order intensity is small (< 15%). The sum of the zero and 1st order intensities corresponds to 90% of the incident intensity for all incidence angles Thus, the diffused light is weak, indicating a satisfactory smoothness of the photoetched grating surface, at this wavelength.

The first order efficiency in TE mode becomes noticeably weaker than in TM mode when the incidence angle is increased. That confirms the electromagnetic nature of the diffraction process on this deep grating at $\lambda = 10.6$ µm.

Gratings with 9.5 µm spacing and 2.0, 2.5 and 4.5 µm depth were characterized similarly at $\lambda = 10.6$ µm. The first order diffraction efficiency is about 80% for the two deeper gratings but markedly decreases (from 80% to 60% following the incidence angle) for the 2.0 µm depth grating. Besides, the profile has no influence on the diffraction efficiencies : the gratings with triangular shape ridges and the same depth show as high efficiencies as the sinusoïdal ones on the first order.

Holographic image recording in GaAs

An holographic image was recorded in a GaAs wafer with the optical set-up shown on the figure 5a. The angle formed by the two incident beams corresponded to a 3 µm spacing allowing details to be recorded with high resolution. The mean laser power density was 40 mW/cm² and the etching time 8s . The reference intensity was seven times higher than the signal one.

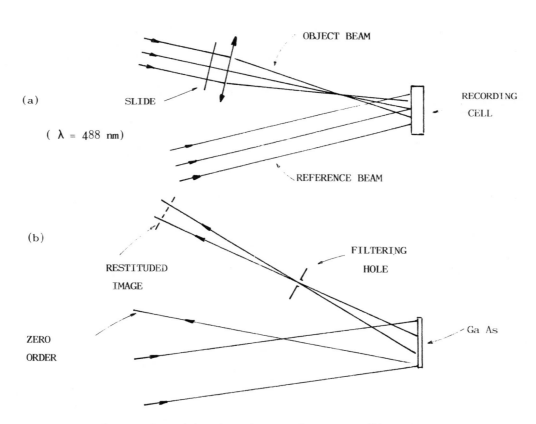

Figure 5. Hologram recording in GaAs (a) and readout configuration (b)

The hologram readout was made in the optical configuration of the figure 5b. A spatial filtering made by the diaphragm allowed an excellent signal/noise ratio to be reached. The restituted image is shown on the figure 6.

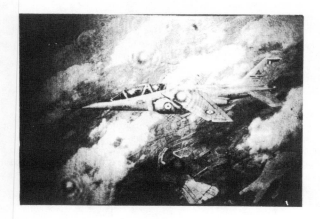

Figure 6. Restituted holographic image

Conclusion

The photoelectrochemical etching technique allows to create reliefs with several microns amplitudes in various semiconductors. It appears well adapted to realize diffractive optical elements with high diffraction efficiencies in the visible and the infrared. Elementary deep gratings were thus engraved in n-doped GaAs, showing first order efficiencies higher than 80% in the infrared, over a large incidence angle range with TM polarization as predicted by the diffraction electromagnetic theory.

The efficiency sensibility to the incident beam polarization may be used or suppressed according to the applications by a judicious choice of the incidence angle. Thus, the photoelectrochemical etching of semiconductors has interesting potential applications in off axis optics.

An holographic image was also recorded by this technique in a GaAs wafer and restituted in the visible with an excellent signal/noise ratio.

References

1 – L.A. D'Asaro et al., IEEE Trans. Electron. Devices ED-25 (1978) 1218
2 – D. Lubzens, Electron. Lett. 13 (1977) 171
3 – F.W. Ostermayer et al., Appl. Phys. Lett. 43 (1983) 642.
4 – D.V. Podlesnik et al., Appl. Phys. Lett. 43 (1983) 1083
    R.M. Lum et al., J. Appl. Phys. 57 (1985) 39.
5 – E.G. Loewen et al., Applied Optics 16 (1977) 2711

Grating interactions in photorefractive materials

Laszlo Solymar

Holography Group, Department of Engineering Science, University of Oxford,
Parks Road, Oxford OX1 3PJ

Abstract

The interaction of two incident plane waves in a photorefractive material is discussed both in the transient and in the stationary case. Preliminary results of a study are presented which solves numerically the transient equations in conjunction with the field equations including optical activity. Comparisons with experimental results show good agreement.

Introduction

Gratings in photorefractive crystals have been the subject of extensive investigations ever since 1968 when the first experiments were performed.[1] The present paper is concerned with the interaction of two symmetrically incident coherent beams in the transmission configuration as shown schematically in Figure 1 where I_{+1} and I_{-1} are the reference and signal beams respectively. The frequency of the reference beam may be slightly shifted by applying a sawtooth voltage to the piezoelectric mirror.

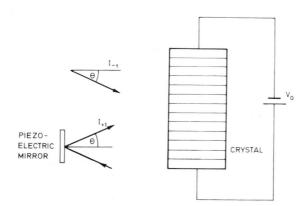

Figure 1. Schematic representation of the illumination of a crystal by two light beams. The frequency of the reference beam may be changed by applying a voltage to the piezoelectric mirror.

A theory that predicted the transfer of power between the beams was first formulated by Staebler and Amodei[2] in terms of coupled wave differential equations. After many attempts which took into account more and more aspects of the rather complex interaction it is now widely accepted that the approach presented by Kukhtarev et al.[3-5] can explain all the experimental results found so far.

Kukhtarev's treatment consists of two parts: firstly, the materials equations which describe the dependence of the refractive index distribution upon the light interference pattern, and secondly, the wave equation in which the effect of the refractive index distribution upon the optical quantities is taken into account.

At thermal equilibrium the photorefractive material is regarded as having a very small dark conductivity, a sizable background of ionised acceptor and donor atoms, and a much larger density of unionised donor atoms. When light is incident some further donor atoms become ionised, the liberated free electrons move under the effect of diffusion and of the applied electric field resulting in a periodically varying net charge density which leads to an electric field and, via the electro-optic effect, to a dielectric grating.

The materials equations

The mathematical relationship between the variables for the one-dimensional case may be written in the following form

$$e \frac{\partial N_D^+}{\partial t} = e \frac{\partial n}{\partial t} + \frac{\partial J}{\partial z} \tag{1}$$

$$\frac{\partial N_D^+}{\partial t} = (\beta_e + sI)(N_D - N_D^+) - \gamma_R n N_D^+ \tag{2}$$

$$J = e\mu n E_s - k_B T \mu \frac{\partial n}{\partial z} \tag{3}$$

$$\frac{d}{dz}(\varepsilon_0 \varepsilon_s E_s) = e(n + N_A^- - N_D^+) \tag{4}$$

where N_D^+ is the density of the ionised donor atoms, n is the density of the electrons, J is the current density, E_s is the static electric field comprising of the applied field and of the space charge, β_e is the rate of thermal generation, s is the cross-section of photo-ionisation, I is the light intensity, N_D is the density of the donor atoms, γ_R is the recombination constant, μ is the mobility, k_B is the Boltzmann constant, T is temperature, ε_0 is the free space permittivity, ε_s is the relative static dielectric constant and N_A^- is the density of ionised acceptor atoms assumed to be constant.

Eqns (1) - (4) are nearly self-explanatory. Eqn (1) is the continuity equation, Eqn (2) contains two terms on the right-hand-side, the first one is the rate of generation (proportional to the density of unionised donor atoms) and the second one is the rate of recombination (proportional both to electron density and ionised donor density). Thus the rate of increase of donor density is equal to the difference between the rate of generation and the rate of recombination. Eqn (3) says simply that the current density is equal to the sum of conduction current density and diffusion current density. Finally, Eqn (4) is Poisson's equation, i.e. relates the net charge density to the rate of change of the electric field.

The light intensity will vary sinusoidally in the z direction. When the two frequencies are slightly different then this interference pattern will travel with a certain velocity v. Hence, in general, the light intensity may be described as

$$I = I_0 + I_1 \cos K (z - vt) \tag{5}$$

where $I_0 = I_{+1} + I_{-1}$, $I_1 = 2(I_{+1} I_{-1})^{\frac{1}{2}}/I_0$, $K = 2\pi/\Lambda$, Λ = grating spacing.

Solution of the materials equations

The differential equations are quite difficult to solve. There have been a number of attempts at various solutions which will be briefly reviewed.

(i) Linearised stationary solution[6]

It is reasonable to assume physically, and it has been shown experimentally, that after a certain time (which may be as long as several seconds) the transients die away and all the material quantities vary at a rate determined by the motion of the fringes. Secondly, one may assume that all the material quantites depend linearly upon the driving term represented by the travelling fringe pattern as expressed by Eqn(5). This means that the $\cos K(z - vt)$ term may be replaced by an $\exp jK(z - vt)$ term and a solution can be written in the form

$$G = G_0 + G_1 \exp jK(z - vt) \tag{6}$$

where G may stand for any of the material quantities. Note that G_0 and G_1 are constants and that $G_1 \ll G_0$ is assumed. Whenever the product of two materials quantities comes up (as for example in Eqn (3) where the charge density is multiplied by the electric field) the cross product of the quantities with subscript 1 is neglected.

(ii) Higher perturbation stationary solution.
The trial solution is attempted in the form

$$G = \sum_{p=0}^{r} \{G_p \exp[jpK(z - vt)] + c.c\} \tag{7}$$

where r is the order of perturbation, c.c. stands for complex conjugate and G represents again any of the variables. Analytical solutions up to the second order have been found[7,8]; beyond that the equations appear to be intractable.

(iii) Phenomenological solution. The experimental results clearly indicate that the available gain is reduced as the input power of the signal beam (to be amplified) increases. This suggests that the modulation of the dielectric constant increases less than linearly with the increase of fringe modulation. Guessing a relationship between these two quantities the experimental results may be matched.[7,8]

(iv) Numerical solution of the nonlinear differential equations. It is also possible to find a numerical solution of Eqns (1) - (4) which makes use of the fact that all the physical quantities must vary periodically as a function of z - vt. In other words, the values of the function and of its gradient must be the same at the beginning and at the end of the period. At sufficiently low modulation we know the initial values from the linearised solution. As the modulation increases and nonlinear effects become important one must make the computer to sweep over a range of initial values and integrates step by step the differential equations until the correct final values are obtained. We are just in the process of trying this method. For stationary patterns and no applied electric field it is relatively easy to find such computer solutions but as the physics and the corresponding mathematics become more complicated the computer time needed to converge to a solution may become excessive.

(v) Linearised transient equations. The trial solution for this case is

$$G = G_0(t) + G_1(t) \exp[jK(z - vt)] \tag{8}$$

where it is assumed again that the spatially varying term is small in comparison with the spatially constant term.

Substituting Eqn (8) for all the relevant physical quantities into Eqns (1)-(4) the following differential equation is obtained[8,9]

$$\frac{\partial E_{1n}}{\partial t_N} + (g - jKv\tau_d)E_{1n} = h\frac{I_1}{I_0} \tag{9}$$

where

$$
\left.
\begin{aligned}
&E_{1n} = \frac{E_1}{E_q}, \quad t_N = \frac{t}{\tau_d}, \quad \tau_d = \frac{\varepsilon_0\varepsilon_s}{e\mu n_0}, \quad n_0 = \frac{sI_0 N_D^-}{\gamma N_A^-} \\[2mm]
&g = \frac{1}{D}\left(1 + \frac{E_t}{E_q} + j\frac{E_0}{E_q}\right), \quad h = \frac{1}{D}\left(-\frac{E_0}{E_q} + j\frac{E_t}{E_q}\right) \\[2mm]
&D = 1 + \frac{E_t}{E_m} + j\frac{E_0}{E_M}, \quad E_T = \frac{KTK_B}{e}, \quad E_M = \frac{\gamma_R N_A^-}{\mu K}, \quad E_q = \frac{eN_A^-}{\varepsilon_0\varepsilon_s K}
\end{aligned}
\right\} \tag{10}
$$

and E_0 is the applied electric field.

Note that I_1 depends on the optical beam intensities I_R and I_s which, in turn, depend on the normalised space charge field E_{1n}. Hence Eqn (9) must be solved in conjunction with the field equations to be presented in the next Section.

The field equations

The differential equation to be solved for the propagation of the optical field vector is the wave equation

$$\nabla \times (\nabla \times \underline{E}) + \frac{1}{c^2}\frac{\partial^2 \underline{D}}{\partial t^2} = 0 \tag{11}$$

where c is the velocity of light, $\underline{D} = \underline{\underline{\varepsilon}}\,\underline{E}$ and $\underline{\underline{\varepsilon}}$ is the dielectric tensor which for BSO (the only material considered in the examples given later) takes the form

$$
\underline{\underline{\varepsilon}} = \varepsilon_0
\begin{pmatrix}
\varepsilon + \Delta\varepsilon & 0 & 0 \\
0 & \varepsilon - \Delta\varepsilon & j\rho/\varepsilon_0 \\
0 & -j\rho/\varepsilon_0 & \varepsilon
\end{pmatrix}
\tag{12}
$$

where $\Delta\varepsilon = -r_{41}\varepsilon_r^2 E_s$, ε_r is the relative dielectric constant at the optical frequencies, r_{41} is the electro-optic coefficient and ρ is the rotatory power which describes optical activity. The relative orientation of the crystal with crystal axes X,Y,Z, the presently used coordinate system x,y,z and the input field vectors are shown in Figure 2.

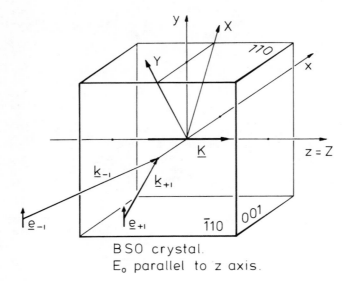

BSO crystal.
E_o parallel to z axis.

Figure 2.   Orientation of the crystal structure relative to the input beams for the BSO
crystal used in the experiments. The input polarisations $\underline{e}_{+1}$ and e_{-1} are in the
y direction.

The solution is assumed in the form

$$\underline{E} = \tfrac{1}{2}[\underline{A}_{+1}(x)\exp j(\omega_{+1}t - \underline{k}_{+1}\cdot r) + \underline{A}_{-1}(x)\exp j(\omega_{-1}t - \underline{k}_{-1}\cdot\underline{r}) + c.c.] \qquad (13)$$

where ω_{+1} and ω_{-1} are the frequencies of the input beams which differ from each other by a
minute amount (of the order of 10 Hz), $\underline{k}_{+1}$ and $\underline{k}_{-1}$ are the input wave vectors and c.c. means
complex conjugate. The amplitude vectors satisfy the normalisation conditions

$$|\underline{A}_{+1}|^2 = I_{+1} \qquad\text{and}\qquad |\underline{A}_{-1}|^2 = I_{-1} \qquad (14)$$

We shall follow now the standard technique of reducing the wave equation to first order
coupled differential equations.[10]   The essential approximations being that the amplitudes
are assumed to be slowly varying functions and higher diffraction orders are neglected.
After a considerable number of arithmetical operations we obtain the two vector differential
equations

$$\frac{d\underline{A}_{+1}}{dx} = \underline{\underline{a}}\,\underline{A}_{+1} + \underline{\underline{b}}\,\underline{A}_{-1} \qquad (15)$$

$$\frac{d\underline{A}_{-1}}{dx} = -\underline{\underline{b}}^{*}\,\underline{A}_{+1} + \underline{\underline{a}}\,\underline{A}_{-1} \qquad (16)$$

where

$$\underline{\underline{a}} = -\frac{\alpha}{\cos\theta}\,\underline{\underline{U}} + \frac{\rho}{\cos\theta}\,\underline{\underline{C}}_1 + j\Gamma E_0\underline{\underline{C}}_2,\ b = j\Gamma E_{1n}^{*}\underline{\underline{C}}_2,$$

$$\underline{\underline{U}} = \begin{pmatrix} 1 & 0 \\ 0 & 1 \end{pmatrix},\ \underline{\underline{C}}_1 = \begin{pmatrix} 0 & 1 \\ -1 & 0 \end{pmatrix},\ \underline{\underline{C}}_2 = \begin{pmatrix} 1 & 0 \\ 0 & 0 \end{pmatrix} \qquad\qquad (17)$$

$$\Gamma = \frac{\pi\varepsilon_r^{3/2} r_{41}}{\lambda\cos\theta}$$

α is the amplitude attenuation coefficient and λ is the free space wavelength.

We still need to express the amplitude of the interference pattern (I_1 in Eqn (5)) with
the aid of the optical vectors which comes to

$$I_1 = \underline{A}_{+1}^{*}\cdot\underline{A}_{-1} \qquad (18)$$

Calculation of beam interaction

For the input conditions shown in Figure 2 when the incident polarisations of the optical fields are in the y direction it is possible to solve the field equations in conjunction with the materials equations. Analytic results for various configurations have been obtained[3-5,7-9,11,12] in the past. It is worth recalling the calculations of Refregier et al.[7-8] which applied both the higher perturbation and the phenomenological approach to obtain good agreement with experimental results concerning all the major effects i.e. dependence of the signal beam amplification on beam ratio, velocity of the fringes and spatial frequency. The absolute amount of amplification was however considerably below that (by about a factor of 6 for the thicker crystal and by a factor of 4 for the thinner crystal) expected from the measured value of the electro-optic coefficient. The discrepancy was probably due to the neglect of two factors, namely attenuation (which means that the fringe velocity will be optimum for only one single value of x) and optical activity (which reduces the interaction between the beams because only the y components of the optical fields are coupled to each other).

Some recent results. We shall show here some preliminary results of calculations[13] which use the linearised transient equations in conjunction with Eqns (15) and (16) to obtain agreement between experimental and theoretical results for the transient amplification at zero fringe velocity.

The amplification of the signal beam as a function of normalised time ($t_N/40$) measured at $\lambda = 514.5$ nm is shown in Figure 3 for two different angles, namely for (a) $\theta = 20°$ and

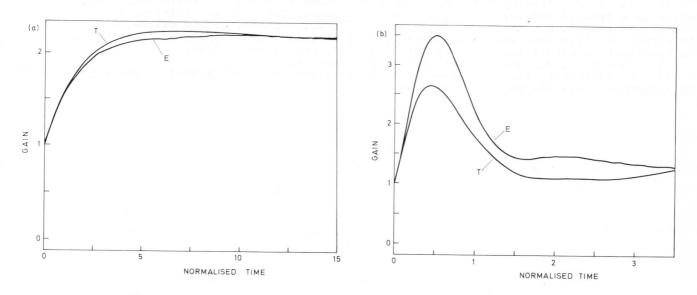

Figure 3. The amplification of the signal beam as a function of normalised time ($t_N/40$) for (a) diffusion dominated and (b) drift dominated regime.

(b) $\theta = 2.2°$ which correspond to the diffusion dominated and drift dominated regimes. The amplification, as usual, is defined as the actual intensity of the signal beam at the output divided by the output signal beam intensity in the absence of the reference beam. The beam ratio is 250 the applied electric field is $E_0 = 7.5$ kV/cm the amplitude attenuation is $\alpha = 0.8$/cm and the length of the crystal is 1 cm. The rotary power ρ is taken[14] as 390°/cm and the rest of the parameters were chosen so as to give the best agreement between the theoretical and experimental results. They are given the values $\mu/(\gamma_R N_A^-) = 1.4 \ 10^7 \mathrm{cm}^2/\mathrm{V}$ $N_A = 0.8 \ 10^{16}/\mathrm{cm}^3$, $r_{41} = 1.7 \ 10^{12}$ m/V. Note that the value of the electro-optic coefficient is about half as much as that given by Pellat-Finet[14] showing that the absolute amplification measured is still lower than the theoretical prediction.

Conclusions

The various methods of solving theoretically the problem of two beam interaction in photorefractive materials have been discussed. The theory, in a form which includes optical activity, has been shown to provide good agreement with experimental results on transient amplification.

References

1. Chen, F. S., La Macchia, J. T. and Fraser, D. B. "Holographic storage in Lithium Niobate," Appl. Phys. Lett., Vol. 13, pp. 223-225, 1968.

2. Staebler, D. L. and Amodei, J. J., "Coupled-Wave Analysis of Holographic Storage in $LiNbO_3$," J. Appl. Phys., Vol. 43, pp. 1042-1049, 1972.

3. Kukhtarev, N., Markov, V. and Odulov, S., "Transient Energy Transfer During Hologram Formation in $LiNbO_3$ in External Electric Field," Opt. Commun., Vol. 23, pp. 338-343.

4. Kukhtarev, N. V., Markov, V. B., Odulov, S. G., Soskin, M. S., and Vinetskii, V. L., "Holographic Storage in Electroopic Crystals. 1. Steady State. 2. Beam Coupling - Light Amplification", Ferroelectrics, Vol. 22, pp. 949-964, 1979.

5. Kukhtarev, N. V., Dovgalenko, G. E. and Starkov, V. N., "Influence of the Optical Activity on Hologram Formation in Photorefractive Crystals," Appl. Phys., Vol. A33, pp. 227-230, 1984.

6. Solymar, L., Wilson, T. and Heaton, J. M. "Space Charge Fields in Photorefractive Materials," Int. J. Electronics, Vol. 57, pp. 125-127, 1984.

7. Refregier, P., Solymar, L., Rajbenbach, H., and Huignard, J. P., "Large signal effects in an optical BSO amplifier," Electron. Lett., Vol. 20, pp. 656-657, 1984.

8. Refregier, P., Solymar, L., Rajbenbach, H., and Huignard, J.P., "Two-beam coupling in photorefractive $Bi_{12}SiO_{20}$ crystals with moving grating: Theory and Experiments," J. Appl. Phys., Vol. 58, pp. 45-57, 1985.

9. Heaton, J. M., "Wave Interactions in Static and Dynamic Volume Holographic Recording Materials," D.Phil. Thesis, University of Oxford, 1985.

10. Kogelnik, H., "Coupled Wave Theory for Thick Hologram Gratings," Bell Syst. Tech. J., Vol. 48, pp. 2909-2947, 1969.

11. Ja, Y. H., "Energy Transfer between Two Beams in Writing a Reflection Volume Hologram in a Dynamic Medium, "Opt. and Quant. Electron., Vol. 14, pp. 574-556, 1982.

12. Heaton, J. M., Mills, P. A., Paige, E. G. S., Solymar, L. and Wilson, T., "Diffraction efficiency and angular selectivity of volume phase holograms recorded in photorefractive materials, " Optica Acta, Vol. 31, pp. 885-901, 1984.

13. Heaton, J. M., and Solymar, L., in preparation.

14. Pellat-Finet, P., "Measurement of the electro-optic coefficient of BSO crystals," Opt. Commun., Vol. 50, pp. 275-280, 1984.

PROGRESS IN HOLOGRAPHIC APPLICATIONS

Volume 600

Session 2

Holographic Optical Elements

Chairmen
J. L. Tribillon
Holo-Laser, France
K. Matsumoto
Canon Incorporated, Japan

The Analysis and Construction of Powered Reflection Holographic Optical Elements (HOEs)

B H Woodcock and A J Kirkham

Pilkington P E Limited,
Glascoed Road, St Asaph, Clwyd, North Wales, LL17 0LL

Abstract

Powered reflection HOES, both spherical and aspherical have been constructed in dichromated gelatin on flat substrates using the back mirror method. Examples of this type of HOE have been investigated inteferometrically and the results compared with theoretical predictions. Some effects of construction geometry and film swelling are discussed.

Introduction

The back reflection technique has been widely used to create reflection holograms, having the advantage that only one beam is used. This forms the reference beam on first passing through the holographic film but becomes the object beam after being reflected or scattered by an object. Denisyuk's[1] method for image holography utilized this principle with great success. It has also been applied to the manufacture of wavelength selective mirrors in head up displays for aircraft[2][3] and in this case can be thought of as a derivative of the Lippmann process.

On account of the need for extremely high resolution, low absorption and freedom from scatter dichromated gelatin has proved superior to even the finest grain Lippman type silver halide emulsions. With the advancement of dichromated gelatin technology, holographic optical elements of acceptable quality can be made in this material.

Where it is necessary to avoid chromatic dispersion holographic mirrors have been made by what amounts to a contact copying process. During exposure the film is held in intimate contact with a mirror of the same curvature such that the standing wave pattern is set up by the interference of the incident and reflected beams conform with the surface. A HOE of this type has no diffractive power, and hence no dispersion, only the geometrical power due to its curvature. Its value lies solely in its photometrical properties as a narrow-band reflector. If a HOE cannot be truly conformal as when an aspherical element is required, diffractive power may be minimized by choosing a spherical substrate with a curvature as close as possible to that of the fringes.

If on the other hand a HOE is to be used in monochromatic light, dispersion is no problem and higher levels of diffractive power can be utilized. This paper considers a method of recording powered elements on flat substrates for possible use in laser systems.

Review of back mirror construction techniques

Figure 1 illustrates three methods of recording a holographic spherical mirror. The simplest method of laying a photosensitive plate on top of a concave spherical mirror and illuminating the combination from the centre of curvature is shown in Figure 1(a). Rays incident on the mirror will be reflected back along their own paths to create a standing wave interference pattern, the fringes of which lie normal to each ray forming a family of concentric spheres. A cross section of these fringes will be recorded in the film to form a hologram whose focal length will be similar to that of the mirror at the wavelength of construction. Such an arrangement has been described by Coleman and Magarinos[4]. For moderate apertures, the effect of refraction by the holographic plate can be neglected provided the plate is thin by comparison with the focal length.

A major problem with this approach is the occurrence of stray recordings due to unwanted reflections at the air to glass surfaces. The preferred approach is to liquid match the inner surfaces wherever possible. The quantity of liquid can be minimized by using an appropriately shaped glass element of the same refractive index to fill the space as in Figure 1(b). The matching liquid and make up glass in this case form a positive lens and modify the focal length of the assembly which acts as a Mangin mirror. The focal length of the resultant HOE is reduced (by a factor equal to the refractive index of the matching medium) with respect to the focal length in air of the construction mirror. The properties of the resultant hologram will depend upon the

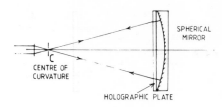

Figure 1(a). Air spaced spherical mirror with flat substrate

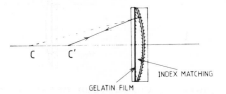

Figure 1(b). Index matched spherical mirror

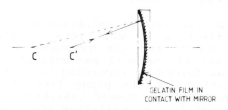

Figure 1(c). Conformal construction with gelatin in contact with mirror

position of the illuminating source. In Figure 1(b) it is assumed that construction takes place from the effective centre of curvature of the assembly, C'.

The source position would have less effect on a conformal holographic mirror such as would be formed by the method shown in Figure 1(c). Here the gelatin film is in contact with the mirror which acts as a constant phase surface regardless of the direction of illumination, but in order to achieve uniform tuning of the hologram (no radial variation in Bragg wavelength) the centre of curvature would again be chosen as the source position. The focal length of the conformal holographic mirror of Figure 3 is identical to that of the construction optics, the hologram behaving in a similar manner to a multilayer dielectric coating since all the recorded fringes are concentric with the surface.

The use of index matching reduces stray recordings to a tolerable level provided a good anti-reflection coating is applied to the front surface. Holographic mirrors of good quality have been manufactured by both these methods at Pilkington P. E. in dichromated gelatin.

Refraction at the glass/air surface of a powered holographic mirror has a significant effect on not only the focal length but also on the spherical aberration. Provided, of course, that a hologram can be constructed exactly in the manner in which it is required to operate, the imagery can be perfect. This is not usually possible using the back mirror method due to aberration of one of the beams by the glass surface at either construction or reconstruction. In many cases the error introduced may be compensated elsewhere in the optical system or may be negligible if the aperture is sufficiently small. If, however, this is not acceptable the HOE may still be made by the back mirror method if a simple means of error compensation can be found. The particular case of a paraboloid mirror is considered in the next section.

Holographic mirrors may in some cases give acceptable optical performance with narrow band phosphors such as P43 but will perform better in monochromatic light. They are ideally suitable for use with a laser system using for example the 514.5nm Argon laser line. This wavelength is particularly convenient for dichromated gelatin work. In this case interferometric standards can apply and diffraction limited quality is desirable.

Holography does not get around the problem of optics flexing and due consideration must be given to the rigidity of the component and the mounting structure. The weight saving resulting from replacing a conventional collimating mirror with a HOE may not therefore be as great as expected, but the potential cost saving could be considerable.

Construction of a holographic paraboloid mirror

In order to investigate the possibilities of back mirror HOE construction, the paraboloid mirror was chosen on account of its general usefulness and availability. It is also a relatively expensive item and so the possibility of making dichromated gelatin copies for monochromatic systems was attractive.

A parabolic HOE could be generated by the classic two beam method Figure 2(a) using a point source and a collimated beam, but unless the physical dimensions were small and the exposure time short, the mechanical stability problems would be considerable. these problems are much reduced by the back mirror method, Figure 2(b), where the holographic plate is in contact with a collimating mirror. Here the point source is shown at the focus of the mirror and serves the dual purpose of illuminating the mirror and providing the reference beam.

Due to the surface reflection problem we have found it necessary to use the index matching technique, discussed earlier, to achieve acceptable holograms. The paraboloid is therefore used as a rear surface (Mangin) mirror. The effective focal length is reduced but the combination does have significant spherical aberration if used as a collimator and a holographic mirror made from a source at its focus would show similar aberration, due to the plane surface of the glass.

In order to reduce this spherical aberration it was necessary to modify the construction geometry and two possibilities were considered:

(i) Illumination from a collimated beam on axis

This is the reverse of construction from the effective focus of the mangin mirror as far as the paraxial rays are concerned, but not exactly so for the marginal rays. The incident beam will

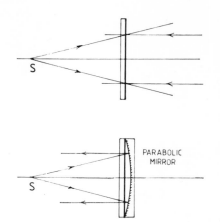

Figure 2. Comparison between (a) the two beam method and (b) the back mirror geometry for axial parabolic HOE construction

in this case be unaberrated since all rays will enter the glass normally. After reflection it will form a spherical wavefront converging on the true focus of the mirror and the fringes caused by interference with the collimated beam will form a set of confocal paraboloids sharing the focal point of the mirror. However, the hologram formed by recording these fringes will not reconstruct a perfect focus due to refraction at the plane front surface. Computation using a Pilkington P. E. optical design programme showed that there was no significant difference between the hologram constructed from a collimated beam and that constructed from a point source at the paraxial focus even for the largest aperture considered (F/2). The reason is that although the ray intersections differ slightly they are almost symmetrical about the normal to the mirror and the fringe slant does not change appreciably.

For simplicity it has been assumed in all computations that the matching fluid, and the gelatin have the same refractive index as the glass, although in practice the variable refractive index of the gelatin may prevent this.

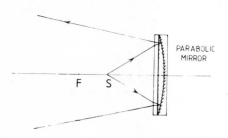

Figure 3. Optimum construction geometry for a parabolic HOE using a back mirror

(ii) Illumination from a point source on axis but not at the focus

The spherical aberration can be improved significantly by changing the point source position and thereby modifying the hologram fringe characteristics. The size of the focal spot was computed as a function of the distance from the mirror of the point source used in construction of the HOE and is shown in Figure 4 for two apertures of mirror. The HOEs were used to focus a collimated beam and it can be seen that there is a sharp minimum at a distance of approximately two thirds of the focal length. The first example, Figure 4(a), is a 31.3 inch focal length collimator of aperture F/3.9. The second example, Figure 4(b), is a 41.9 inch focal length F/2.6 collimator. For the smaller apertures the HOE will focus a collimated beam to a spot with a geometrical radius close to that of the Airy Disc. For the larger aperture higher order aberrations are present which reduce the image quality.

The effect of aperture on theoretical performance is shown in Figure 5, where the minimum geometrical focal spot size using optimum construction geometry is plotted against hologram radius, for the case of the 41.9 inch holographic collimator. Figure 5 also shows the radius of the Airy Disc and the geometric spot size which would be obtained from a conventional spherical mirror used as a collimator. It can be seen that the geometrical focal spot from the hologram is smaller than the Airy Disc for apertures of less than F/3.5. The spherical mirror similarly requires apertures of less than F/8.

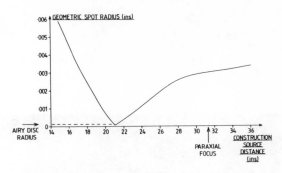

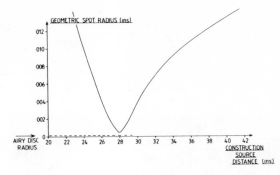

Figure 4. Focal spot size as a function of source distance at construction
(a) A 31.3 inch focal length 4 inch radius HOE (F/3.9) (b) A 41.6 inch focal length 8 inch radius HOE (F/2.6)

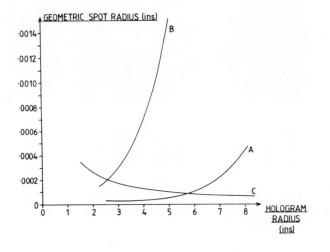

Figure 5. Focal spot size as a function of source distance at construction
A : A parabolic HOE constructed using optimum source distance
B : A conventional spherical mirror
C : The Airy Disc

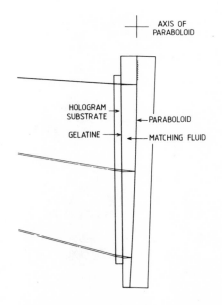

Figure 6. Construction of an off-axis HOE

Figure 7. Layout of test interferometer

These calculations were carried out for mirrors and HOEs used on-axis. The off-axis case can be evaluated by considering the aperture of the equivalent on-axis mirror.

Experiments have been carried out on two paraboloid mirrors. The first was an F/6 axial mirror with 48 inch focal length in air, whilst the second was an off-axis mirror of 64 inch focal length and 6 inches aperture, whose centre was 5 inches off-axis. The latter can be regarded as a section of an F/4 mirror. Construction of the off-axis hologram is shown in detail in Figure 6. Both direct (object beam) and reflected (reference beam) rays are shown in this diagram.

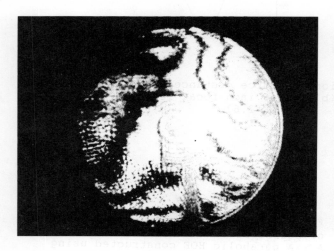

Figure 8. Interferogram of axial HOE

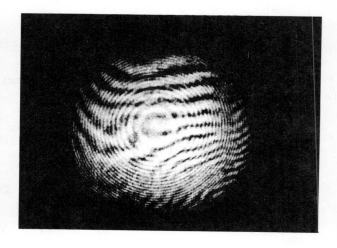

Figure 9. Interferogram of off-axis HOE

Holograms were constructed in dichromated gelatin on glass plates 10mm thickness, this being the minimum thickness considered to have sufficient stiffness over an 8 inch diameter.

Each was exposed at 514.5nm and processed to give a maximum reflectivity at the same wavelength. They were then tested on the interferometer shown in Figure 7 for the off-axis case. This required the HOE to be used twice, first to collimate the light and then to refocus it after reflection at a plane mirror, thereby doubling the effect of the wavefront error. The interferometer was adjusted so that the refocused spot was superimposed upon the primary focus at the surface of the beamsplitter.

Figure 8 shows the interferogram of an F/3.9 HOE constructed using the F/6 paraboloid mirror, showing less than two wavelengths of error over this aperture. From the irregular nature of the fringes it is likely that some of the wavefront aberration was caused by random errors and did not represent the best which could be achieved. Results for the 8 inch aperture off-axis HOE are shown in Figure 9. Here the wavefront error is considerably greater, as would be expected from the prediction of Figure 5 for an F/2.6 (full aperture) HOE. Figure 10 shows the computed blur spot diagrams for the two cases. In the case of the axial F/3.9 collimator, the geometrical spot diagram is 0.8 times the corresponding Airy disc radius, so the collimator is close to being diffraction-limited on axis. The shape of the off-axis spot, Figure 10(b), is asymmetrical and suggests the presence of coma. However comparison with Figure 10(c) showing the

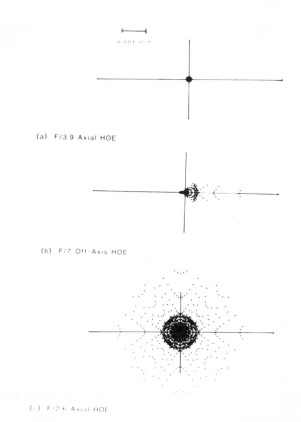

(a) F/3.9 Axial HOE

(b) F/7 Off-Axis HOE

(c) F/2.6 Axial HOE

Figure 10. Computed focal spot diagrams

aberration for the equivalent full aperture on-axis mirror shows this is in fact part of a high-order spherical aberration pattern. The appearance of horizontal and vertical symmetry in Figure 10(c) is not significant as it results from the use of a rectangular array of points in the entrance pupil.

As shown in Figure 4(b), for the off-axis collimator it is not possible to achieve a geometrical spot size comparable to the Airy disc, using a parabolic construction mirror. Near-perfect imagery is, however theoretically achievable using a construction mirror of hyperbolic profile with further sixth and eighth order figuring terms; such a mirror is obviously not a standard catalogue item.

Although the results quoted are for HOEs used at the wavelength of construction, similar performance can be achieved at other wavelengths by controlling the swelling of the gelatin provided the source distance is re-optimized for the wavelength required.

The HOE once completed can be used as a back mirror itself to enable copies to be made, if due allowance for the extra glass thickness has been taken into account in its construction.

Conclusions

The back mirror method of HOE construction has advantages in terms of stability and ease of construction. Refractive index matching improves the optical quantity but leads to spherical aberration when a powered mirror is recorded in a flat element and used as a collimator. This can be explained in terms of geometrical optics and is due to refraction at the air/glass surface. It has been shown that this aberration can be minimized by suitable choice of construction geometry and that near diffraction-limited performance can be achieved for useful apertures around F/4, in monochromatic light. Such powered reflection HOEs could find application in laser systems.

Acknowledgements

The authors wish to express their thanks to the Directors of Pilkington P. E. Limited for permission to present this paper and also to S. S. Duncan, D. M. Ring and others for their valuable assistance.

References

1. Denisyuk, Yu. N., Optics and Spectroscopy, Vol 15, pp279-284. 1963.
2. Vallance, C. H., Proc. SPIE, Vol 399, pp15-25. 1983.
3. Woodcock, Proc. SPIE, Vol 399, pp333-338. 1983.
4. Coleman, D. J. and Magarinos , J., Applied Optics, Vol 20, pp2600-2601. 1981.

Transmission holographic optical elements in dichromated gelatin

R. W. Evans

Pilkington Brothers PLC, R&D Laboratories, Lathom, Ormskirk, Lancs., England.

Abstract

Holographic Optical Elements operating on light by diffraction are beginning to find a role in optics complementary to those of mirrors and lenses, that is reflective and refractive optics. Holographic elements working in either transmission or reflection can be made.

Introduction

If a holographic material is to be suitable for high quality optical elements it must have adequate spatial resolution, suitable spectral response and sensitivity, be a phase material with sufficient controllable refractive index modulation, produce holograms of very low scatter and absorption, give stable performance, have good film forming properties, and be able to produce holograms of sufficiently good uniformity and reproducibility to meet the required performance specification.

Many laboratories are carrying out research into a wide range of holographic materials, and a number of very interesting materials are under development. However dichromated gelatin is currently established as the best, proven material for high quality holographic optical elements for the most demanding applications.

Techniques for making reflection holographic optical elements in dichromated gelatin have been developed into a viable industrial production process and a manufacturing facility has been set up for this purpose by Pilkington P.E. These H.O.E.s are now finding use in applications such as combiner plates in aircraft head-up-displays, narrow band reflection filters, contrast enhancement filters, tunable wavelength selective filters and image holograms.

Dichromated gelatin can produce high quality, stable, holographic optical elements with a wide range of characteristics manufactured to very tight tolerances.

Reflective H.O.E.s

A head-up-display is an optical system for projecting information displayed on a cathode ray tube into a pilot's line of sight as he looks out of his aircraft. The C.R.T. information is superimposed on the view of the outside world by reflection from a semi reflecting glass combiner plate. If a narrow bandwidth reflection holographic optical element is used as the combiner plate in conjunction with a C.R.T. phosphor emitting in a narrow spectral band, then high reflectivity of the displayed image can be combined with high transmission of light from the outside world away from the reflection band.

Some new head-up-display systems make use of holographic optical elements with broad bandwidths, but reduced reflectivity to maintain a high integrated visible transmission of light from the outside world.

Narrow band reflection filters are being made which are particularly effective for use with lasers. Filters with half height bandwidths upwards from less than 10 nm can be made which transmit less than 0.01% of the peak reflective wavelength.

Holograms can be used as contrast enhancement filters. Such a filter may comprise several holograms made with the required bandwidth and tuned to reflect away sunlight in the spectral bands outside the emission bands of C.R.T. phosphors so improving display contrast.

Dichromated gelatin holograms can be made to operate in the near infra-red and a demultiplexing device for communications applications is being developed which reflects in a narrow bandwidth, but the wavelength reflected varies along the length of the filter from 1.25 to 1.6 microns.

Image holograms are now also being replicated into dichromated gelatin to give bright images of controllable colour.

Transmission H.O.E.s

Dichromated gelatin is now being developed for use in making transmission H.O.E.s for which a range of practical applications is emerging. Holographic optical elements can be made which closely match the predictions of planar hologram theory for the diffraction efficiencies in the various orders of diffraction. Similarly transmission holographic optical elements operating by Bragg diffraction have diffraction efficiencies approaching the theoretical predictions.

The light intensities in the various orders of a planar transmission holographic grating are described by the squares of the Bessel functions of the first kind of order corresponding to the order of diffraction.

By looking at the curves of the Bessel functions it can be seen that the intensity in the zero order, the two first orders, and two second orders of diffraction can be made approximately equal. If two such gratings are positioned in series and mounted orthogonally it should be possible to produce a 5 x 5 array of light beams of approximately equal intensity from a single input beam. According to this model the intensities of all the beams should lie within about ±20% of the mean.

A holographic construction system was used to generate fringes of 10 micron spacing. Holograms have been made in 20 micron thick films and the refractive index modulation carefully controlled.

Good control of the intensity in the zero, first, and second orders has been achieved and pairs of holograms have been sealed together so as to act to produce 5 x 5 arrays. The intensities of each of the diffracted beams has been measured and fairly close agreement with the theoretical model has been seen. All the intensities lie within +25% of the mean, and the standard deviation is +18%. Improvements in the uniformity may well be achievable, from further development work.

Bragg effects and non-linearities in the exposure processing schedules will clearly influence the performance achieved.

This kind of device has potential applications in communications systems, optical computing and parallel processing.

Another important application of transmission holographic optical elements is laser scanners for reading bar codes. It is desirable to use them with very low power lasers, either helium neon or laser diodes, for reasons of safety and low cost. Consequently optimum performance requires the use of very high diffraction efficiency optical elements, for which dichromated gelatin is well suited.

Holographic laser scanners are usually made in the form of facets or segments around the circumference of a disc. The disc is rotated at high speeds to scan and focus an array of lines so that at least one line will scan the bar code to be read. The light reflected from the bar code is usually refocussed by the hologram facet onto a detector.

Anything up to twenty or more holographic facets may be put on the disc depending on the volume of space over which it is required to scan.

The more sophisticated scanners employ transmission holograms with slanted fringes. To meet the Bragg conditions, this necessitates processing a disc with up to around twenty holographic facets on it so as to achieve a very high degree of control of film thickness, not only from facet to facet, but within each individual facet. Dichromated gelatin technology has been developed to meet just these sort of stringent tolerances and this together with the high diffraction efficiency which can be achieved indicates that dichromated gelatin can be used for large volume production.

Acknowledgement

This paper is published with the permission of the Directors of Pilkington Brothers PLC and Mr. A. S. Robinson, Director of Group Research and Development.

Progress in diffractive Optics for H.U.D

Jean-Blaise MIGOZZI

Service Technologie Optique – THOMSON-CSF AVG
52 Rue Guynemer 92115 ISSY LES MOULINEAUX
FRANCE

Abstract

Thanks to numerous progress particulary in chemical technology, computer automatic design, Computer Generated Holograms (C.G.H), and industrial means, diffractive optics can be used widely.

Introduction

Several companies in the world have developped their own technologies in diffrative optics, mainly for display applications and particularly for the head-up display. The company Thomson-CSF has not escaped this common rule.

We have however tackled the building of holograms as a general problem the problem of manufacturing optical components.

Thanks to the progress we have made for ten years we can now apply holography to numerous problems, which are much wider than the head-up display field.

Progress in Chemical Technology

- decrease of the scattered light rate. In this domain, our progress (we have diminished this rate from 10 to 1) enables us to take into account all the faced applications.

- raise of sensitivity. We have improved this by seven in six years. We have experienced that the maximum size of an hologram is restricted by the exposure time and by the quality of automatic regulation of registening waves.

We are now in a position to produce holograms which sizes are 50 cm x 50 cm.

- mastery and adaptation of the Bragg's angle (or the efficient wavelength) and of the angular (or the spectral) band width.

These two parameters are of great importance for all the structures using the turning - back of beams by the means of holography - as for example holograms by double reflexion (see figure 1).

- Moreover, our latest studies regarding new photopolymeres seem very attractive.

Progress in design of holographic lens

1) Difficulties of the holographic computing

When computing the motion of beams in a conventional optical system, the beam deflection caused by an optical interface depends only on the features of this optical interface (radius of curvature, index rate, impact point).

In an holographic system, the beam diflexion at a determined point depends also on the two registering beams which have reached this point.

The determination of these beams is rather long, as it is a non-deterministic problem, which demands numerous iterations (see figure n° 2).

These iterations are all the more complicated and long as the registering systems are more complex. It is often the case as registering systems are often manufactured one by one and used in a laboratory.

2) Our solutions

Our main progress in this field have consisted in setting aside this procedure while separating the design work into two parts :

- computing the holographic combination,
- computing the registering system.

A - Computing the holographic combination

Our theoritical studies have led us to represent the holographic diflexion function by some Chebichev and Legendre's polynomial series.

The holographic diflexion function is not defined through registering beams.

As a consequence, the computing of beam diflexion doesn't depend, as in the conventional optical systems, on the impact point of the beam on the optical interface.

The motion of beams through the optical system is done at the same time as the computing of accurate derivatives.

The optimisation algorithm which is used looks like a P.S.D (pseudo second derivative) method. But this method has been considerably improved and adapted to the Chebichev and Legendre's representation.

B - Computing the registering system

Once the computing of the holographic combination is performed, we have to determine the registering system which will be used to build the computed holograms. At this step of the work, these ones are defined only through the polynomial representation of their holographic diflexion and through the features of the glass support.

The selected method and the software which has been developped enable us to choose among 3 possibilities.

1 - Optimisation of a registering system which includes only conventional optical parts

This is an iterative method. It consists in computing a registering system which will later build an hologram. During that, the difference between the hologram achieved by this registering system by and the aimed computed hologram must be reduced.

2 - Determination of a registering system including optical parts which are previously designed and a C.G.H. This method is a completely deterministic method : once the beams through the registering system, the computing of this C.G.H is done.

3 - Determination of a mixed registering system

(i.e including both conventional optical parts and a C.G.H). This method is a mixture of the above mentionned methods : the remaining error due to the first method is compensated by the application of the second method.

Thanks to the software we have developped, we are now in a position to meet all the requirements regarding the holographic and conventional optics. These computing of requirements come from our company, as well as from other companies with which we have gone into partnership.

Computer Generated Holograms (C.G.H)

When a high optical quality is necessary, conventional optical parts cannot often supply registering waves with the required accuracy. Moreover, these waves may be quite complex.

The only solution is C.G.H. At the moment, we are able to produce C.G.H with 8000 fringes and which sizes are 50 x 50 mm.

Progress in industrial means

Thomson-CSF has equipped one of its works with large industrial means, including a dust-free and air-conditioned room.

Several millions dollars have been spent to set up a man production works. Its production capacity has been scheduled for much larger needs than our own neads. That is why we can also meet other companies needs. We have also widened our activity to the manufacturing of holographic optical parts.

Consequences for the H.U.D

All these progress have been applied to the head-up display. In comparison with our first prototypes, we have reached satisfactory results in all the major fields :

- size of the eye-box : it has been multiplied by 2.

- number of lenses in the relay lens : it has been divided by 2.
- weight of lenses in the relay-lens : it has been divided by 2.

Figure : 1

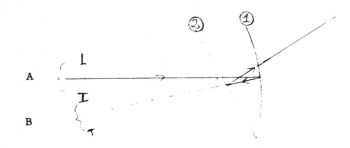

Holograms by : double reflexion

A is the efficiency aera of hologram 1

B is the efficiency aera of hologram 2

A must be close to B in order to reduce off ascis on 1

A must be separated from B to avoid reflexion by 2 of rays from A.

Figure : 2

registering lens

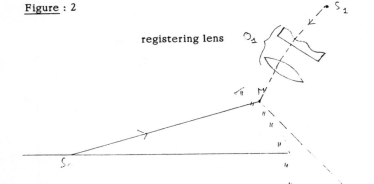

registering lens

Holographic computing

A ray from S_O reach the hologram on M the problem is to determine wich rays from S_1 (across O_1) and from S_2 (across O_2) have registred the hologram in M.

ACHROMATIC DISPLAY HOLOGRAMS IN DICHROMATED GELATIN

Harry Owen and Andrew E. Hurst

Pilkington P.E. Ltd, Glascoed Road, St. Asaph, Clwyd, LL17 OLL, U.K.

Abstract

This paper looks at the production of achromatic reflection holograms in dichromated gelatin. By using a double exposure technique we can produce two reflection bands in the same emulsion with complementary dominant wavelengths. This results in the colour mixture being close to the achromatic point on a chromaticity diagram.

Introduction

White light reflection holograms with good image depth generally appear to be monochromatic to the viewer. The replay colour can be tuned to the laser construction wavelength (real colour) or tuned to any other wavelength within the visible spectrum (pseudocolour).

In this paper we look at how twin reflection bands can be produced by double exposing the dichromated gelatin emulsion to the argon blue line at 457nm and the argon green line at 514nm. If the two reflection bands are tuned so that they have complementary dominant wavelengths the resulting colour mixture will be within the achromatic zone on a chromaticity diagram.

Dichromated Gelatin Technology

Dichromated gelatin (DCG) can be used to produce image holograms with very high diffraction efficiencies (>99%), excellent resolution, low levels of optical scatter and spectral tuning over a wide wavelength range. Bright blue, green, yellow, orange and red display holograms in dichromated gelatin where exhibited by Pilkington P.E. earlier this year at the SPIE 1985 Los Angeles Technical Symposium on Optical and Electro-Optical Engineering. To consistently produce good quality holograms in DCG it is necessary to use clean rooms supplied with air which is tightly controlled for temperature and relative humidity. Each stage of the process needs to be carefully controlled if good reproducability is to be obtained i.e. process solutions need to be filtered, temperature and pH stabilised. High powered argon ion lasers are used to keep exposure times as short as possible while well isolated optical tables are used to minimise vibration problems.

To produce a hologram with a specific performance a process schedule needs to be generated by identifying suitable values for the parameters listed below:-

Process parameters
Gelatin Film Thickness
Gelatin Film Hardness
Concentration of sensitizer
Exposure Geometry
Exposure Wavelength
Exposure Level
Process Temperature

Suitable values are derived from our understanding of the relations between the process parameters and the holographic properties. Listed below are the primary relationships between the process parameters and the holographic properties.

Gelatin film thickness
Increasing the film thickness will reduce the spectral bandwidth and provide greater image depth.

Gelatin film hardness
Increasing the film hardness will reduce the level of optical scatter.

Concentration of sensitizer
Increasing the level of the sensitizer will reduce the fringe spacing and the spectral tuning position will move towards the blue end of the visible spectrum.

Exposure geometry
Increasing the angle of incidence away from the normal moves the spectral tuning position towards the red end of the spectrum.

Exposure wavelength
Decreasing exposure wavelength will cause the spectral tuning position to move towards the blue end of the spectrum

Exposure level
Increasing the exposure level will increase the diffraction efficiency and cause the spectral tuning position to move towards the blue end of the spectrum.

Process temperature
Increasing the process temperature will increase the diffraction efficiency and the spectral bandwidth resulting in increased replay brightness.

To produce two different but balanced reflection bands in the same film a double exposure technique was developed. Account has to be taken of the sensitivity of the DCG film to the different construction wavelengths as well as the overall exposure level.

Double Exposure Technique

The blue line (457nm) and the green line (514nm) of an argon ion laser were used to produce the two reflection bands. To achieve the correct exposure balance between the two construction beams, holographic mirror samples were produced using a diverging beam incident upon a sensitized film in contact with a plane mirror, the incident and reflected beams interfere to set up the required fringe pattern.

These holographic mirrors were evaluated so that the spectral tuning position, spectral bandwidth and diffraction efficiency could be calculated and used to optimise the process.

Holographic mirror samples with:-

i)   Blue and green reflection bands.
ii)   Blue and yellow reflection bands.
iii) Green and yellow reflection bands

were manufactured and assessed. The holographic properties of these samples are outlined in Table 1.

SAMPLE	BAND	SPECTRAL POSITION	SPECTRAL BANDWIDTH	DIFFRACTION EFFICIENCY
BLUE/GREEN	1st	462	11	97%
	2nd	519	16	99%
BLUE/YELLOW	1st	465	30	99%
	2nd	576	40	99%
GREEN/YELLOW	1st	519	18	97%
	2nd	585	26	99%

Table 1

Spectral traces of samples i) and iii) are reproduced below in Figures 1 and 2.

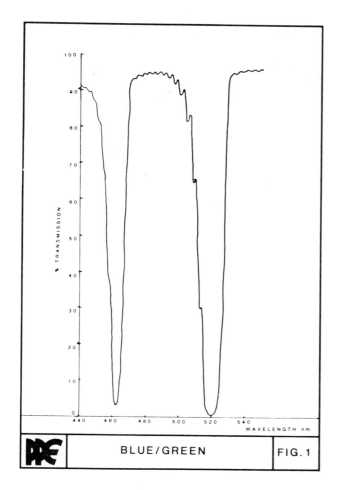

Figure 1

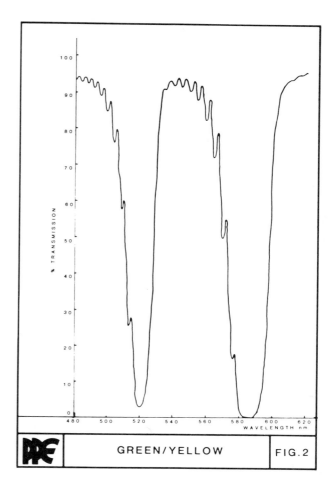

Figure 2

An analysis of the data indicates that the double exposure technique and proprietary tuning methods can achieve a suitable level of performance. Diffraction efficiencies of over 95% in each reflection band will certainly provide bright replay characteristics.

At the correct viewing angle the blue/yellow filter produces achromatic reflection properties that can be viewed using a colour chart.

Definition of Colour

Diffraction efficiency, spectral tuning position and spectral bandwidth describe closely the characteristics and shape of the reflection band of the holographic mirror samples. These values are normally for measurements made at normal incidence in a suitable spectrometer.

Spectral bandwidth
Defined as the width of the reflection band at 50% transmittance.

Spectral tuning
Defined as the point midway between the edges of the spectral bandwidth at 50% transmittance.

Diffraction efficiency
Defined as the reflectivity at the peak wavelength.

For display holograms new parameters need to be defined. The brightness and replay colour should take into account the type of light source and the spectral response curve of the human eye as well as the holographic performance.

We used the "Handbook of Colorimetry" compiled by A.C. Hardy at the Massachusetts Institute of Technology (Copyright 1936) for the basis of interpretation of the data obtained from the evaluation of our display holograms.

Measurements were made using a Spectra Pritchard Photometer Model 1980A located some 1180mm from the centre of the hologram.

Light from a Wotan Quartz halogen lamp was used to illuminate the hologram. The light source was located 1948mm from the centre of the hologram at an angle 31° from the plane of the hologram.

A Wotan lamp was used because it is probably the most widely used light source for holographic lighting purposes and it is reasonably close to the illuminant C point on a chromaticity diagram. The photometer is initially calibrated against a std illuminant A source before it is used to calculate the tristimulus values X, Y & Z for each display hologram. Since the tristimulus value for Y corresponds exactly with the visibility curve for a normal eye it is a direct measurement of the perceived brightness of the hologram. By using the tristimulus values X,Y & Z we can define three new quantities x,y & z. The trichromatic coefficients define the quality of the colour. Normally only x and y are used to specify the chromaticity of a sample. By plotting the position of x and y onto a chromaticity diagram two additional parameters can be calculated.

Dominant Wavelength and Purity

The dominant wavelength of a colour is the wavelength associated with the point on the spectrum focus intersected by a straight line drawn through the sample point from the illuminant or achromatic point.

The purity is a measure of how strongly the dominant wavelength contributes to the colour of the sample. The purity is calculated by comparing the relative distances of the sample point and the corresponding spectrum point from the illuminant point.

Specifying the colour of holograms in terms of brightness, dominant wavelength and purity is useful because they closely relate to the three psychological attributes of brilliance, hue and saturation. The chromaticity diagram is extremely useful when 2 colours are added together because the resulting colour is always located on the line joining the points of the individual colours.

Display Holograms

A set of Denisyuk type display holograms with single and double reflection bands were produced for colour evaluation. The object was a machined aluminium disc with a depth of about 6-8mm. This type of object was used so that the double exposure technique developed using an aluminium mirror as the object could still be used with the minimum of modification. Holograms with single reflection bands were tuned to give blue, green and yellow replay characteristics. Holograms with double reflection bands were tuned to give blue/green and blue/yellow replay characteristics.

Optical measurements were carried out using the Spectra Pritchard photometer as outlined earlier. The optical data calculated from the measurements is listed in table 2.

SAMPLE	TRICHROMATIC COEFFICIENTS		DOMINANT WAVELENGTH	PURITY %
	x	y		
BLUE	0.189	0.123	464nm	70
GREEN	0.238	0.625	548nm	94
YELLOW	0.505	0.458	582nm	90
BLUE/GREEN	0.191	0.340	493nm	42
BLUE/YELLOW	0.499	0.419	586nm	78

Table 2

The trichromatic coefficients x and y have been plotted on chromaticity diagrams (see Figures 3 & 4).

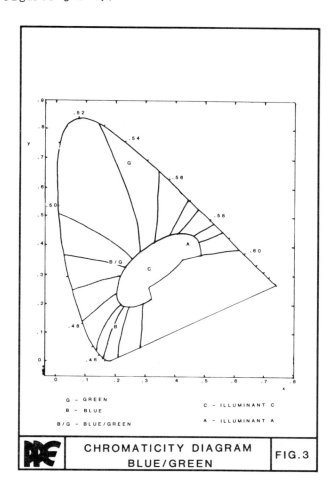

Figure 3

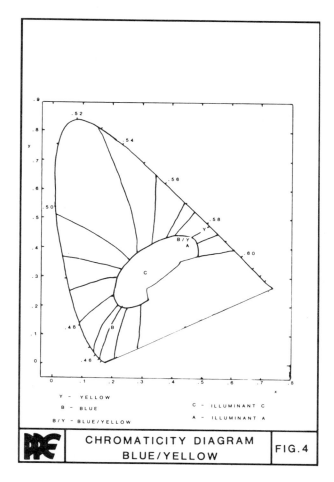

Figure 4

The colour coordinates of the single blue, single green and double blue/green holograms are plotted on Figure 3. The blue/green point is located in between the single blue and green test points as expected.

Because of the spectral values of the blue and green reflection bands it is not possible to produce an achromatic mixture. However since we have produced a real colour blue/green hologram it is a useful step in the right direction for obtaining full colour holography.

The colour coordinates of the single blue, single yellow and double blue/yellow holograms are plotted on Figure 4. The blue/yellow point is located between the single blue and yellow test points just within the achromatic region of the chromaticity diagram close to the illuminant A position. Visually a metallic appearance is produced but with a slight yellowish tinge. The proportions of the yellow and blue components need to be better balanced to produce a mixture point closer to the illuminant C position.

<u>Conclusion</u>

We have demonstrated that twin reflection bands with complementary spectral tuning and high diffraction efficiencies can be produced in a DCG film. Consolidation of this process to take into account correct proportioning of the spectral bandwidths will enable good quality achromatic reflection holograms to be commercially available in the near future.

Acknowledgements

The author wishes to thank the directors of Pilkington P.E. Ltd for permission to present this paper.

References

1.   Owen H., 'Display Holograms in Dichromated Gelatin', The Second International Symposium on Display Holography (1985).

Holographic Embossing at Polaroid:
The Polaform Process

James J. Cowan and W. Dennis Slafer

Research Laboratories, Polaroid Corporation
750 Main St., Cambridge, MA., 02139

ABSTRACT

Embossing of replica holograms at the Polaroid Corporation is being done in two major areas: crossed grating arrays for development of new types of photographic films and holographic optical elements; and the production of white-light viewable display holograms of various types for many diverse applications.

INTRODUCTION

The Holographic Research Laboratories at Polaroid are involved in many diverse areas of research and development of current interest in holography. One of these, and the subject of the present paper, is the mass replication of holograms by means of embossing (the "Polaform" process). Other areas of interest include holographic imaging research with emphasis on stereograms using primarily silver halide recording materials; and research and production of volume phase type reflection holograms in a new photopolymer material.

The Polaform process is a holographic embossing technique that consists of the following major steps: recording of a holographic interference pattern in photoresist; formation of a master metal replica of the photoresist pattern by electroplating; and use of the metal master or a metal replica to repeatedly emboss this pattern into long sheets of plastic. In certain cases, there is a fourth step involving metallizing and die cutting of the plastic sheet.

The types of holographic patterns that are recorded are linear and crossed grating arrays for use in certain types of holographic optical elements and for the ordering of photographic grains into low noise film systems; and display holograms, including both production and experimental work with the image plane, rainbow, stereogram, and surface plasmon types.

PHOTORESIST RECORDING

Recordings are done in a positive-working photoresist, in which exposed areas are preferentially etched away upon development over non-exposed areas. Assuming conditions of linearity, the developed surface of the photoresist will be a surface relief profile whose depth is directly proportional to the incident interference intensity. Linear development is achieved, for example, by use of preexposure or with certain types and concentrations of developers. The use of other developers will lead to a nonlinear response, in which the least exposed areas etch very little with respect to the most exposed areas. In general, the nonlinear response is preferred for the crossed grating deep hole patterns required by the photographic system because of the better definition of the holes, while the linear response is preferred for the display holograms because of the reduction of noise. Since photoresist is sensitive only in the short wavelength end of the spectrum, the recordings considered here are made either at the 442 nm line of the He-Cd laser or at the 458 nm line of the argon ion laser.

CROSSED GRATING ARRAYS

Three types of crossed grating arrays have been made: A square pattern, consisting of two linear gratings, exposed sequentially at ninety degrees to each other; a hexagonal (or honeycomb) pattern, consisting of a single simultaneous three-beam exposure, with each of the sources arranged at the apexes of an equilateral triangle (see Figure 1); and a quad (or egg-crate) pattern, consisting of a single simultaneous four-beam exposure, with each of the sources arranged at the corners of a square. The first of these arrays yields a two-dimensional checkerboard-like etched surface of hills and valleys. With the nonlinear response, the hills etch little and appear flat, and the valleys resemble parabolic shaped cups. Thus the surface area consisting of cups is about half of the total area. The latter two configurations yield close-packed honeycomb and square structures consisting of parabolic shaped cups that occupy practically all of the available surface area. Figure 2 shows the theoretical intensity curves for the hexagonal array. Also the intensity ratio from the center to the edge of each cup in the simultaneously exposed arrays is larger than in the sequentially exposed one, so the etched hole depth is always larger for these cases. For the positioning of photographic grains, both close packed and deep structures are desirable, so the simultaneously exposed arrays are preferable for this purpose. The mathematical treatment of the crossed grating array patterns has been given in References 1-3.

DISPLAY HOLOGRAPHY

     A two step procedure is used for display holograms. In the first step a large glass plate is coated with a thin layer of photoresist. A hologram is made in this plate consisting of light reflected from some object interfering with a collimated reference beam from a large diameter lens. After development the plate is repositioned but reversed, so that a real 1:1 magnified image is formed when illuminated with the collimated beam. A second plate coated with photoresist is placed at the focus of this image, the light from which now constitutes the object beam, and another collimated reference beam is brought in to interfere with this light, making an image plane hologram. Figure 3 shows the recording configuration for this process. If the aperture on the large lens is restricted to a narrow slit in the second exposure, the result will be a rainbow hologram. If the real image is focused onto one face of a prism onto which has been coated a layer of photoresist on top of a thin silver layer, and a reference beam is brought into the prism from behind at greater than the critical angle, stimulating a surface mode, then a surface plasmon hologram will be formed. A more detailed description of surface plasmon holography has been given in References 4 and 5.

REPLICATION AND EMBOSSING

     The next step in the replication process is to produce a nickel plate from the pattern formed in photoresist. The developed photoresist plate is coated with a vacuum evaporated layer of silver, making it electrically conductive, and is immersed in an electroplating bath consisting of an electrolyte and a nickel anode. With the resist plate acting as the cathode, a layer of nickel is then plated onto the resist surface. After a sufficiently thick layer has been produced, the resist plate is stripped away, and the nickel plate can be used in the next step of the process, which is embossing. Figure 4 is a micrograph of a nickel replica of a deep hexagonal pattern. The plate can be fashioned into a cylindrical shape that makes it suitable for mounting onto a machine that allows for continuous embossing into plastic. The plastic must be softened by either heat, pressure, solvent or some combination of these. Some types of plastic that are suitable are vinyl, polycarbonate, mylar, or cellulose esters. The nickel plate has a surface relief profile that is the mirror image of the original pattern formed in photoresist. The pattern that is impressed into plastic is thus the same as the photoresist pattern. If the mirror image is desired, however, it is possible to extend the metal replication process one step further, so that a daughter nickel plate is formed from the master nickel plate. The embossing is then done with the daughter plate. In general, replication is easier and the embossed relief profile is more faithful to the original for shallow patterns than for deep ones. Figure 5 shows a replica of a shallow hexagonal pattern. Pulling and tearing that might be expected for some sharp edged patterns is lessened here because of the rounded bottom edges that result from the holographic process. Figure 6 illustrates a section of plastic embossed with a crossed grating pattern that has been illuminated with a white-light point source that displays the characteristic spectra.

APPLICATIONS

     Embossed crosed grating patterns can be used directly in a subsequent process of aligning photographic grains. There are two methods for doing this. The first involves coating fully formed and sensitized photographic grains directly into the cups. The second is a multi-step process that involves first coating the cups with an unsensitized small grain emulsion, then coalescing these grains into larger grains, and finally sensitizing the larger grains. Figure 7 is a micrograph of a close-packed hexagonal pattern coated with the fine grained emulsion. Figure 8 shows a time series of the growth of grains by coalescence, under the action of a solvent (KBr) at an elevated temperature (90° C.). It has been shown that the granularity noise perceived in an image is related to the randomness of positioning of the photographic grains[5]. In areas of maximum exposure density, for example, granularity noise is maximum for a completely random arrangement of grains, but becomes significantly reduced when the grains are regularly arrayed. A detailed treatment of our research on this subject has been recently reported[7-9], and some of the more extensive photographic results shall soon be published.

If the embossed mirror image of these patterns is produced, i.e., embossed plastic posts (or domes) instead of cups, then the array can be used as a microlens. A deep pattern of micrometer sized domes has an application as a selective solar window, and a shallow pattern of millimeter sized domes can be used as a fly's eye lens for three dimensional integral photography. Figures 4 and 5 are examples of deep and shallow replica structures that would be appropriate for these purposes. A detailed description of the honeycomb microlens has been given in Reference 3.

Plastic sheet that is embossed with display holograms is coated with a vacuum evaporated layer of aluminum to increase the efficiency. Careful consideration must be given to control of the original etch depth in photoresist, because the efficiency depends not only on the etch depth, but also on the type of dielectric overcoating. Since the display holograms are viewed through the clear plastic base, a smaller etch depth is required for an equivalent efficiency than for a metal layer without an overcoating layer or for a transmission hologram without a metal layer at all. Underetching leads to dim holograms, but overetching leads to burnout.

Most of the holographic crossed grating patterns considered above are used in nonimaging situations, and thus the flatness of the substrate is not of paramount importance. Embossings have been done successfully into plastic sheets of three mil (0.0762 mm) thickness. For imaging elements, such as the fly's eye array, embossing would have to be done into a thicker, more rigid substrate. Although the display holograms are embossed into the thinner three mil sheet, they are always die cut and mounted by pressure sensitive adhesive onto thick plastic or paper substrates. The quality of the adhesive is important here to minimize "orange peel" or mottle effects.

Some recent display holograms that have been made by the techniques described above are shown in the remaining figures. Figures 9 and 10 show holograms of an object combined with a holographic crossed grating pattern. The former of these has been described in Reference 4, and the latter was used to commemorate the 25th anniversary of the laser at the 1985 CLEO conference[10]. Figures 11 through 13 combine a front illuminated view of an object with a diffusing background using two different reference viewing angles. The first of these was used on the cover of the stockholders' annual report for 1985 of the Mountain Bell Telephone Company. With the second, the H1 plate was recorded on silver halide using red laser light, and the H2 was recorded onto photoresist using blue laser light[11]. The resulting hologram appeared on the cover of the summer 1985 issue of Artforum magazine. Figures 14 and 15 are of holograms for which the objects were specifically made for artistic content, through the help of a resident artist. These holograms were all intended to have a satisfactory degree of viewability under adverse lighting conditions, especially fluorescent lighting, but like most white-light viewable holograms, they appear best when seen under bright, point source illumination. Alternate versions of several of these images have been made using rainbow and full aperture techniques.

ACKNOWLEDGEMENTS

The authors wish to thank Francis Levitre for his extensive help with the laboratory procedures of the embossing group; Deborah Dunham, our "resident artist", for conceiving of and building the models used in making these holograms; Charles Giles, for doing the nickel electroforming; and Manny Chiuve, Ralph Burpee, and Virgil Andrews, for doing the electron micrographs.

REFERENCES

1. J. J. Cowan, "The Recording and Large Scale Replication of Holographic Crossed Grating Arrays using Multiple Beam Interferometry" in International Conference on the Application, Theory, and Fabrication of Periodic Structures, Diffraction Gratings, and Moire Phenomena II, Jeremy M. Lerner, ed., Proc. SPIE 503, 120 (1984).

2.   J. J. Cowan, U. S. Patent 4,496,216 (Jan. 29, 1985); J. J. Cowan, International Patent Application PCT 84/02781, published July 19, 1984, claiming U. S. filing date of Dec. 30, 1982.

3.   J. J. Cowan, "Holographic Honeycomb Microlens", Optical Engineering, 24(5), 796-802 (September/October 1985).

4.   J. J. Cowan, "The Newport Button: The Large Scale Replication of Combined Three- and Two-Dimensional Holographic Images" in Optics in Entertainment II, Chris Outwater, ed., Proc. SPIE 462, 20 (1984).

5.   J. J. Cowan, "Surface Plasmon Holography", AIP Conf. Proc. No. 65, Optics in Four Dimensions - 1980, p. 415.

6.   J. C. Dainty and R. Shaw, Image Science, Academic Press, New York (1974), p. 102.

7.   V. K. Walworth, A. B. Holland, and W. D. Slafer, "Thin Layer Coalescence of Silver Halides", Proc. SPSE 38th Annual Conference, Atlantic City, N. J., May 12-16, 1985.

8.   W. D. Slafer, J. J. Cowan, M. Fitzgerald, and V. K. Walworth, "Investigation of Arrayed Silver Halide Grains", Proc. SPSE 38th Annual Conference, Atlantic City, N. J., May 12-16, 1985.

9.   J. J. Cowan and W. D. Slafer, "The Recording and Large Scale Replication of Crossed Holographic Grating Arrays using Multiple Beam Interferometry", Proc. SPSE Annual Conference, Atlantic City, N. J., May 12-16, 1985.

10. Conference on Lasers and Electro-Optics, Baltimore, Md., May 21-24, 1985. The hologram and crystal paperweight were sponsored jointly by Polaroid, the Newport Corporation, and Crystal Impressions Division of Precision Optical Co.

11. This hologram was a joint production of Polaroid and the Museum of Holography, New York City. The H1 hologram was made by Dan Schweitzer of the Museum of Holography.

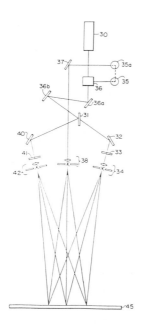
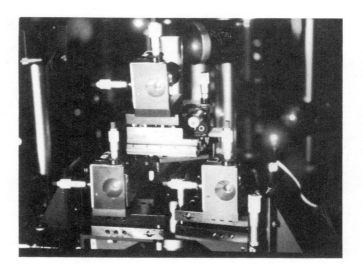

Figure 1. Recording apparatus for hexagonal pattern; left, top view; right, array of sources as seen from the target.

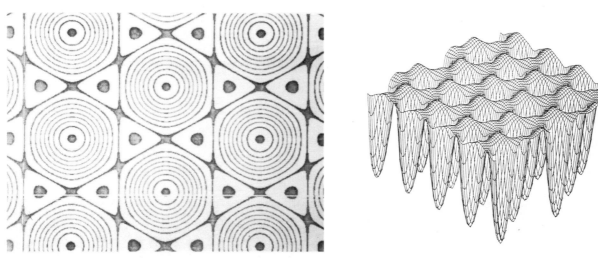

Figure 2. Theoretical equal intensity contours for hexagonal pattern; left, top view; right, isometric view.

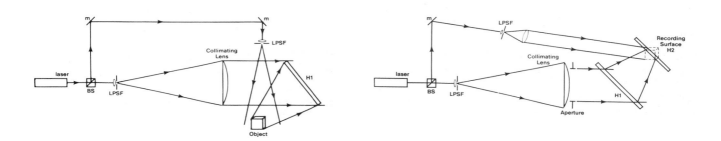

Figure 3. Recording configuration for display holograms; left, first step; right, second step.

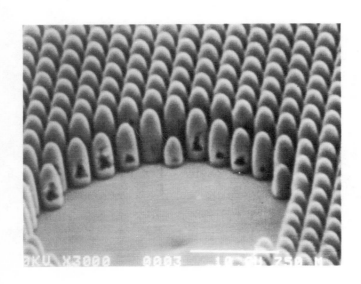 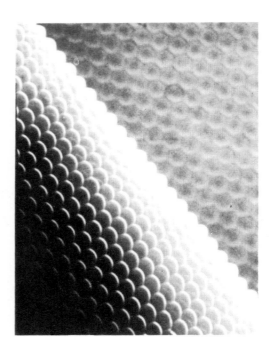

Figure 4. Nickel replica of deep hexagonal pattern.   Figure 5. Replica of shallow hexagonal pattern - edge view.

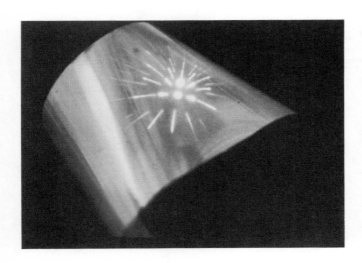 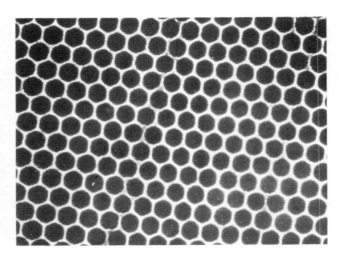

Figure 6. Plastic sheet embossed with crossed grating pattern.   Figure 7. Fine grained emulsion coated into embossed hexagonal cups.

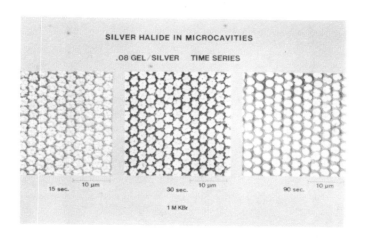

Figure 8. Coalescence of silver halide grains in hexagonal microcavities.

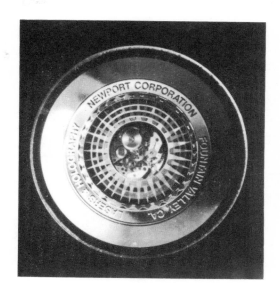

Figure 9. Newport paperweight; combined hologram and crossed grating pattern.

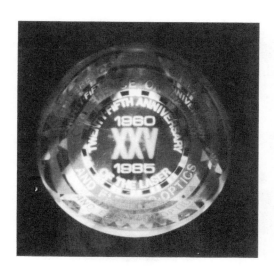

Figure 10. CLEO paperweight; combined hologram and crossed grating pattern.

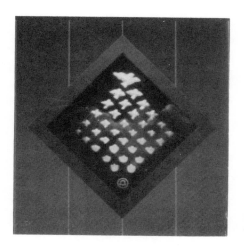

Figure 11. Mountain Bell hologram.

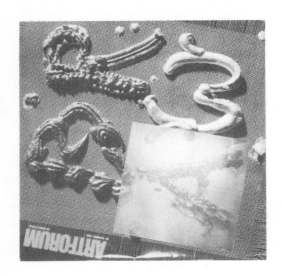

Figure 12. Artforum hologram.

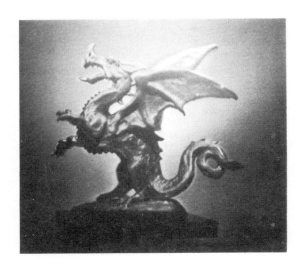

Figure 13. Dragon hologram.

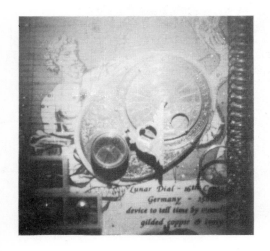

Figure 14. Lunar dial hologram.

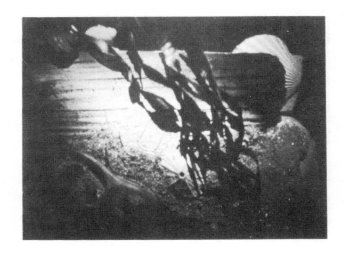

Figure 15. Seascape hologram.

Image blurring in display holograms and in holographic optical elements

A. A. Ward, J. C. W. Newell and L. Solymar

Holography Group, Department of Engineering Science, University of Oxford,
Parks Road, Oxford, OX1 3PJ

Abstract

A review is given of image blurring mechanisms in reflection and transmission holograms for both monochromatic and white-light replay. A theoretical model based on ray-tracing and locally-planar grating 2-beam coupled-wave theory is used to analyse dispersion blurring in white-light holograms as a function of wavelength in terms of the angular blur of an image-point seen by an observer. Methods of minimizing the blur are given, and the significant reduction achieved by recording reflection holograms with a tilt is explained and illustrated by experimental results. The use of a thick recording material is proposed as a method of producing full-parallax transmission holograms which can be replayed with white-light without dispersion compensation, and some preliminary results are given. The theoretical model used can also be applied to the analysis of the imaging properties of holographic optical elements.

1. Introduction

Display holography represents a radical departure from conventional imaging systems. As far as information content is concerned it is vastly superior to its predecessors, but the same cannot be said for fidelity of reproduction. Holographic images will differ from the original objects in a number of ways; the aim of the present paper is to consider one particular aspect of this lack of faithful reproduction, namely blurring.

In 2-Dimensional imaging (e.g. photography) blurring refers to the way an object point is optically projected onto a 2-D image plane in real time by a lens system, and specifically to the size (and shape) of the image of each object point on the fixed image plane. The situation in holography is more complex in that there are two things to consider: the holographically reconstructed 3-D wavefront, and the observer's viewing system, which images a portion of the former into a 2-D image which may be blurred in the same way as in the real time 2-D imaging case; the blurring seen by the observer will depend upon the numerical aperture of his imaging system, its focal length, its position and orientation in the space in front of the hologram - all of which are variable - as well as on the quality of reconstruction of the wavefronts by the hologram. In moving around, or by using stereo vision, the observer will also perceive some 3-dimensional nature to any observed blur: for each object point he will perceive some form of 3-D fuzzy blob, but this will not necessarily be fixed in space - it will appear to change with viewing position.

Thus we cannot describe a blurred image in a hologram as if it were a fixed blurred object, or directly in terms of errors in the wavefront reconstruction; we must always refer to the observer's position and viewing system. However, we can simplify the situation by supposing that the viewing system has a very small aperture and so a large depth of focus, which will give us the blur due to errors in the wavefront reconstruction alone, although we still need to specify the observer's position. This situation corresponds closely to viewing a hologram with a human eye.

One may distinguish three mechanisms which cause blurring in display holograms:

a) Dispersion

When a hologram is replayed with a white or other broadband light source, the various component wavelengths are in general diffracted at different angles (and at different intensities), so that the image will appear spectrally dispersed and blurred in one direction. The range of wavelengths which are diffracted at significant intensity depends on the Bragg selectivity of the grating at each point on the hologram, which is a function of the grating thickness and period. The degree of dispersion then depends on the grating orientation, which varies with position on the hologram and with object-point position. The degree of dispersion is thus determined at the recording stage, and can be minimized by methods described later.

b) Replay source size

The angle of diffraction of a ray leaving a hologram is a function of its angle of incidence, so that if a hologram is reconstructed with a source of finite angular extent (as measured at the hologram), each point of the original object will appear angularly blurred (for a white or monochromatic source). The degree of blurring will depend on the intensity profile of the source, and upon the angular selectivity of the hologram, which is a function of the grating period and orientation at each point on the hologram. In effect, each image point is a diminished 3-D image of the light source imaged in a holographic lens or mirror formed by an object point and the reference source at recording; blurring will increase with increasing distance of the image point from the plane of the hologram, it is very small for points very close to the hologram plane.

c) Geometric distortion

If the replay reference source is not in exactly the same position relative to the hologram as the recording reference source was, or if the replay wavelength is not the same (i.e. if for white-light replay the emulsion thickness or refractive index has changed), then the re-constructed image will be geometrically distorted and delocalized[1], i.e. the apparent position of any image point will vary with viewing position and direction. Thus if the observer's viewing aperture is relatively large, the image will appear blurred. This type of blurring is, however, not caused exclusively by the peculiarities of wavefront reconstruction; it is also present when an object is viewed through relatively thick glass or under water. The two effects are of course compounded when a hologram has a relatively thick substrate. It should be emphasized that for a very small aperture viewing lens there is no blurring in this case.

Of these three blurring mechanisms, dispersion is usually the most significant in white-light holography, and is the main topic of this paper; it is the reason why reflection holograms normally give better results with white-light reconstruction than do transmission holograms, and is the reason why special techniques normally have to be used to achieve satisfactory results from transmission holograms if they are to be replayed with white light – such as the use of dispersion compensation[2] or parallax restriction as used in rainbow holography[3]. However, we demonstrate that transmission holograms can in fact give similar results to reflection holograms if they are made in a sufficiently thick recording material.

Blurring due to replaying a hologram with an extended source is the next most significant mechanism since practical white-light sources must be of finite size if they are to have finite intensity. A compromise has to be chosen between brightness and source size, but display holograms often suffer severe blurring due to a bad choice of illumination lamp: particularly those with semi-diffuse reflectors; the only decent source for holograms of more than a few centimeters depth is a low-voltage quartz-halogen lamp mounted in high-quality slide projector optics at least 2m from the hologram.

Blurring arising from the presence of geometric distortions is not usually significant for holograms viewed with the human eye (except in large-scale projection holograms where, invariably, only a very approximate conjugate reference source is used), but will become relatively significant if a hologram is replayed with an 'ideal' light source (i.e. a monochromatic point-source), especially if the wavelength is not the same as at recording.

The three blurring effects will of course compound each other, and some improvement will always be gained by reducing any one of them, although a sensible balance of efforts must be chosen, taking into account the discrimination of the observer's viewing optics.

Plate 1(a) is a photograph of a reflection hologram of our test object replayed with a near ideal source (actually a fltered high-pressure mercury lamp without optics), which thus has minimal blur. The object was 100mm behind the hologram plate. Plates 1(b) to 1(e) illustrate various degrees of blurring due to dispersion, when source-size blurring has been minimized by use of the light source mentioned above (approx. 7.5mrad). These plates are referred to in more detail below. Plate 1(f) illustrates the effect of increasing the source size by removing the focussing lens from the projector; comparing with plate 1(e), it can be seen that even this gives a significant deterioration.

2. Theoretical Modelling

We are going to use a ray-tracing analysis which assumes the hologram grating layer to be very thin compared to its other dimensions and to the distances of all object points and reference sources, but thick compared to the wavelength of light. Thus rays are angularly deviated by Bragg diffraction at the hologram plane, but not laterally deviated (except by the hologram substrate).

The object is modelled as an array of independent point sources, and the hologram grating is modelled as a 2-D array of locally-planar volume gratings formed by interference between object rays and a reference ray at each point in the hologram plane: rays are treated as wide parallel beams once inside the recording layer, and the hologram grating will exhibit wavelength and angular selectivity at replay. Diffraction other than the Bragg diffraction of the hologram is disregarded, and the gratings formed by different object points are assumed to be independent of each other for the purposes of calculating ray directions.

The above model has been used successfully to model geometric distortions in display holograms to a high degree of accuracy; it is such that if a hologram is replayed with an ideal source (point, monochromatic) at the correct wavelength and position, wavefront reconstruction will be 'perfect' and there will be no blurring except for that due to the presence of a thick substrate.

In practice, hologram gratings are between 5 and 100µm thick on a 1-6mm thick glass substrate, so the above assumptions are normally good approximations. The model allows for the effects of a glass substrate, assuming this to be flat, parallel-sided, homogeneous and rigid. This assumption is likely to be the limiting factor in the accuracy of the model, in addition to the possibility of lateral distortion of the grating layer in the case of thicker gelatin layers, as we found in our experiments with thick transmission holograms described below.

Calculations were made with reference to a coordinate system based on a typical overhead-referenced display hologram: the origin is defined to be coincident with the centre of the hologram, with the x-y (z=0) plane coincident with the grating plane; the y-axis is upward. the x-axis horizontal to the right, and the z-axis toward the observer. Thus an overhead reference source would normally be in the y-z (x=0) plane, at a +ve z position for a reflection hologram, or a -ve position for a transmission hologram. To minimize blurring, overhead-referenced reflection holograms are normally made with a vertical tilt (see below), in which case the observer's horizontal plane will be tilted relative to the z-x plane, requiring a simple coordinate transformation.

To illustrate more clearly the essential features, a two-dimensional simplification is made in the analysis by taking the reference source, viewing point and object points to be in the y-z (x=0) plane, and considering rays in this plane only; extension to the general, 3-D, case is given briefly.

Figure 1 illustrates the theoretical modelling in 2-D of the recording of a hologram, illustrating three example rays from a single (arbitrary) object point intersecting rays from a reference source at three points on the hologram. Reflection reference rays are shown as solid lines, and transmission reference rays as dashed.

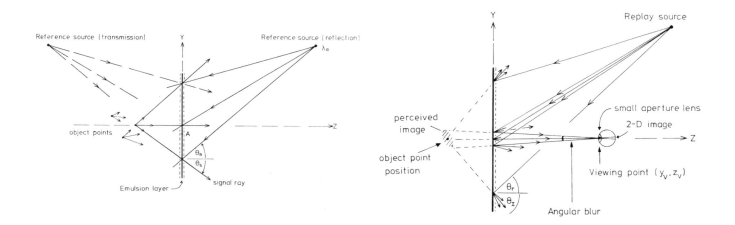

Fig. 1: 2-D ray diagram of hologram recording geometry.

Fig. 2: 2-D ray diagram of hologram replay.

Figure 2 illustrates the theoretical modelling in 2-D of the replay of a reflection hologram, considering the image of object point (0, -50mm) seen by an observer with an approximately zero-aperture imaging lens at some point in front of the hologram. If the reference source is either white or extended, rays from more than one point on the hologram will pass through the viewing point (y_v, z_v), and the observer will see a blurred image of the object point. For this zero-aperture case, we need only specify the angles of image-forming rays, and so describe the blurring in terms of the angular extent of rays forming the image of any particular object point.

3. Blurring due to dispersion in holograms replayed with white light

In this section we describe blurring in white-light reflection or transmission holograms resulting only from the finite wavelength selectivity of the hologram; we assume that the replay source is very small and is in the same position as the recording reference source. The general form of the blurring in this case is illustrated in figure 3, which is a schematic diagram of the 2-D view seen by an observer looking at a hologram of an array of six object points. The spot above the hologram is the position of the replay source for a transmission hologram, or the position of its reflection in the hologram plane for a reflection hologram.

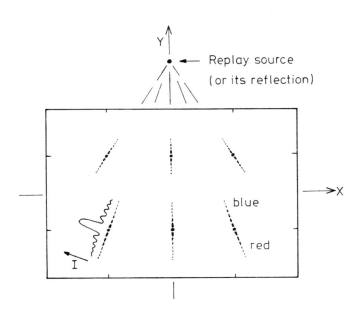

Fig. 3: General form of the dispersion blurring in a
white-light hologram of six point-objects.

The images of the object points are chromatically dispersed along lines which extend from the object point toward the reference spot, with the blue end upward. Each line will have an intensity profile illustrated by the curve to the side of the figure, with maximum brightness normally at the recording wavelength and object- point position. The width of the intensity profile is a function of object position and of the wavelength selectivity of the hologram; normally it will be narrow for reflection holograms and very wide for transmission holograms. A qualitative analysis of this blurring is given below, confining analysis at first to the 2-D model (i.e. the centre two points in fig. 3), and to describing the blur as an angular deviation from the correct direction of the image point.

3.1 Calculation of dispersion blurring

The calculation is in two parts: first the angular blur is found as a function of wavelength which is independent of the actual wavelength selectivity of the hologram, then the superimposed intensity profile is calculated using the results of coupled wave theory.

Angular blur as a function of wavelength. Referring to figure 2; for one particular object point we need to find the apparent direction, θ_V, of the image-forming ray which passes through the viewing point as a function of wavelength, λ. This is determined by the replay reference ray angle and the grating period and angle at each point on the hologram, the latter being determined by the recording geometry and wavelength:

At recording (see figure 1) the grating is formed by interference between a reference ray at an incidence angle of θ_R, and a signal ray from the chosen object point at an angle of incidence of θ_S. This is illustrated by the vector diagram of figure 4: (a) for a reflection hologram, and (b) for a transmission hologram. (θ_R is defined to be between ±90°, rather than between 90° and 270° in the reflection case; this results in a ± sign being introduced into the expressions below which should be taken as + for transmission and - for reflection.) The diagram relates to point A on the hologram in fig. 1. The reference ray is identified by wave-vector $\overline{\rho}_R$, and the signal ray by wave-vector $\overline{\sigma}$; the magnitude of these vectors is $2\pi/\lambda_R$, where λ_R is the recording wavelength, and their directions are θ_R and θ_S. Inside the emulsion layer (refractive index n_e) the waves become $\overline{\rho}_R'$ and $\overline{\sigma}'$

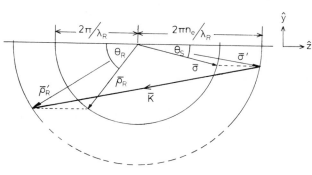

(a) Reflection

(b) Transmission

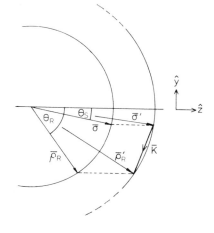

Fig. 4: Recording - wave-vector diagrams

$$\bar{\rho}_R' = \frac{2\pi}{\lambda_R} \left(\pm\sin\theta_R \, \hat{y} \pm (n_e^2 - \sin^2\theta_R)^{\frac{1}{2}} \hat{z} \right) \tag{1}$$

$$\bar{\sigma}' = \frac{2\pi}{\lambda_R} \left(\sin\theta_S \, \hat{y} + (n_e^2 - \sin^2\theta_S)^{\frac{1}{2}} \hat{z} \right) \tag{2}$$

where $\hat{y}$ and $\hat{z}$ are the coordinate unit vectors
so that $|\bar{\rho}_R'| = |\bar{\sigma}'| = 2\pi n_e/\lambda_R$

The resulting grating vector, $\bar{K}$, is given by

$$\bar{K} = \bar{\rho}_R' - \bar{\sigma}' \tag{3}$$

At replay, the diffraction of the incident replay wave by the grating is illustrated by the vector diagram of figure 5: (a) for reflection and (b) for transmission. The reference source is white, so there are many wavelengths λ_r, although only three are illustrated.

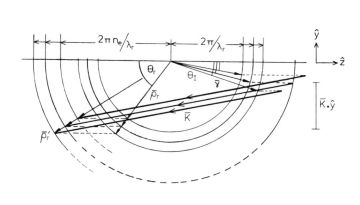

(a) Reflection

(b) Transmission

Fig. 5: White-light replay - wave-vector diagrams

The incident reference rays are identified by wave-vectors $\bar{\rho}_r$, of magnitude $2\pi/\lambda_r$ and angle θ_r. These are refracted into the emulsion layer to become waves $\bar{\rho}_r'$, which are then diffracted by the grating $\bar{K}$.

The diffracted wave vectors $\bar{\gamma}$ are given by satisfying two conditions[3]:

(a) $|\bar{\gamma}| = |\bar{\rho}_r| = 2\pi/\lambda_r$ (4)

and   (b) $\bar{\gamma}.\hat{y} = (\bar{\rho}_r - \bar{K}).\hat{y} = \pm\dfrac{2\pi}{\lambda_r} \sin\theta_r - \dfrac{2\pi}{\lambda_R} (\pm \sin\theta_R - \sin\theta_S)$ (5)

as shown in the diagram. The image-forming ray leaves the hologram at the angle θ_I, which is different for each wavelength component, λ_r. It can be seen from the construction of fig. 5 that for a given wavelength range the spread of image-ray angles θ_I increases with increasing slant of the grating (i.e. with $\bar{K}.\hat{y}$, the component of the grating vector parallel to the boundary, which varies with position on the hologram.); this spread tends to zero at the point on the hologram where the grating is unslanted for a reflection hologram ($\theta_R = -\theta_S$), or where $\bar{K}=0$ for a transmission hologram ($\theta_R = \theta_S$) (but in this case the hologram is no longer a volume grating and multiple diffraction orders will appear).

If we have a fixed viewing point (y_v, z_v), then for a diffracted ray to be seen originating from the point on the hologram $(y,0)$, the image-ray direction θ_I, must be equal to the viewing direction, θ_V:

$$\theta_I = \theta_V = \tan^{-1}((y_v - y)/z_v)$$ (6)

This will fix the wavelength of the observed ray; it can be shown from equations 1-6 that

$$\lambda_r = \lambda_R \left[\frac{\pm \sin\theta_r + \sin\theta_V}{\pm \sin\theta_R + \sin\theta_S}\right].$$ (7)

Since λ_r must be positive, it can be seen from the above expression that there are two limits between which the image of any particular object point may be visible:
1) The viewing angle at which $(\pm\sin\theta_r + \sin\theta_V) = 0$
   i.e. along the observer's line of sight to the reference source or its reflection. This limit obviously changes with viewing position.
2) The point on the hologram where $(\pm \sin\theta_R + \sin\theta_S) = 0$
   i.e. the point where $\theta_S = -\theta_R$ (reflection) or $\theta_S = \theta_R$ (transmission), which has already been mentioned as the point where dispersion is zero. This point is not a function of viewing position.
Furthermore, as limit (1) is approached, $\lambda_r \to 0$, and as limit (2) is approached, $\lambda_r \to \infty$.

These limits are illustrated in figure 6, in which a transmission replay source is shown in the same position as the reflection of a reflection replay source.

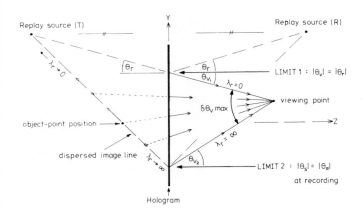

Fig. 6: Angular dispersion limits.

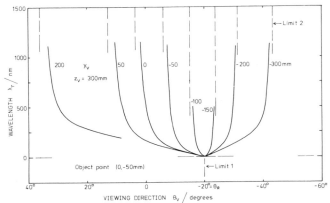

Fig. 7: Blur as a function of viewing position.

It can be shown that the apparent positions in depth of the dispersed images of the object point are along a line from the reference source (or its reflection)(where $\lambda_r = 0$) through the object-point position (where $\lambda_r = \lambda_R$) to the hologram (where $\lambda_r = \infty$).

It can be seen that the maximum possible blur defined in fig. 6 will in general be a function of object-point position, reference source position and viewing-point position, and can easily be found by drawing fig. 6 for the appropriate parameter values.

The blur can generally be reduced by
a) moving the viewing-point away from the hologram,
b) moving the object-point closer to the hologram,
c) reducing the reference beam angle.

There is zero blurring of any image point which lies on a line between the observer's eye and the reflection of the reference source; the two limits coincide in this case.

As an example, figure 7 shows a set of curves of θ_v vs λ_r for the image of object point $(0,-50)$, as seen from five viewing positions 300mm from the hologram; the reference is a parallel beam at $\theta_r = -20°$.

If we wish to consider object points or viewing points which are not in the y-z (x=0) plane, we must extend the ray-tracing analysis to 3-D: Equations 3,4,5 are still valid, and we need only add the condition on the diffracted wave, $\bar{\gamma}$, that

$$(c) \quad \bar{\gamma}.\hat{x} = (\bar{\rho}_r - \bar{K}).\hat{x}$$

(8)

There is still only one ray seen by the observer for each wavelength component, and it can be shown that the image is still dispersed along the line from the replay source (or its reflection) through the object point to the hologram, as in fig. 6, with the same two limits. The dispersed image will now of course appear at an angle, as illustrated in fig. 3.

Angular blur intensity. Having found the maximum possible angular blur, we now need to calculate the relative intensities of the dispersed image rays, so as to model the actual visible angular blur; this will be a function of the wavelength selectivity of the hologram, which is proportional to the grating thickness normalized to its local period.

We use the results of Kogelnik[5] for the amplitude of the diffracted wave in a uniform plane grating, inserting the value of λ_r from equation (7) for each value of θ_r at each point on the hologram. Since these are only two-wave solutions, they cannot be used to model the actual intensities of diffracted rays in a hologram of an extended object. However, the width of the off-Bragg intensity profile given by these solutions (close to a sinc curve) is almost independent of intensity (for low efficiency), and it is only this information that is required to calculate the extent of the angular blur: we assume only that this width is given correctly for each component wave as a function of angle and wavelength; this can be checked by experiment. The intensity profile and wavelength of a blurred image point as a function of viewing angle is plotted in figure 8 for both reflection and transmission holograms of equivalent geometry (i.e. the transmission reference source is in the same place as the reflection of the reflection reference source); the emulsion thickness is 5μm, the object point is (0,-100mm), the viewing point is (0,300mm), and the reference is a distant source at 30°. For a given geometry, the width of these curves reduces with increasing grating thickness.

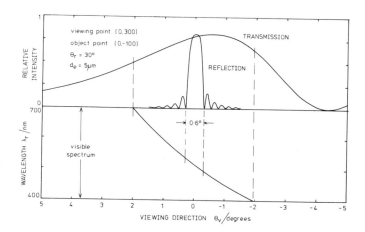

Fig. 8: Angular blur intensity and wavelength profiles.

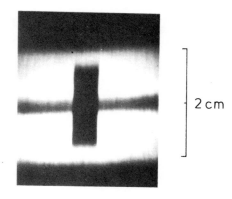

Fig. 9: Photograph of a thick transmission hologram replayed with white light.

Figure 8 clearly illustrates the reason why transmission holograms made with conventional 5μm thick recording plates (Agfa 8E56 or 8E75 silver-halide emulsions) cannot be replayed with white light unless either dispersion compensation is used[2], or they are rainbow projection holograms[3] (where the vertical dispersion is made unimportant at the expense of losing vertical parallax). Dispersion compensation is in effect equivalent to using a reference source at $\theta_R = 0°$ to minimize the angular blur as described above, while retaining the volume grating characteristics of the hologram (i.e. only one diffraction order).

However, if a sufficiently thick recording material is used inconjunction with a high reference beam angle, a transmission hologram can be recorded which exhibits similar selectivity to a conventional reflection hologram. This is demonstrated in figure 9, which is a photograph of a transmission hologram recorded in a dichromated gelatin layer 60μm thick, with a reference beam angle of 70° and replayed with white light without dispersion compensation. The object (a back-lit diffusing screen) was 60mm behind the hologram plane.

Having calculated the intensity profile as a function of wavelength from coupled wave theory, the actual observed brightness will be given by multiplying this by the replay source spectral curve and by the human eye response curve if appropriate.

3.2   Reduction of dispersion in reflection holograms

The angular blur for a reflection hologram illustrated in fig. 8 is excessive even for human-eye viewing (0.6° ≡ 4.2mm at 400mm distance), as illustrated by plate 1(b) which is a photograph of a test object hologram of equivalent geometry to fig. 8, recorded on Agfa 8E56 and illuminated with a small white-light source. The vertical dispersion of the image is clearly seen as a loss of resolution of horizontal lines, and as a spread of the bright spots, in which it is possible to see the side-lobe structure. The blur is actually slightly worse than would be seen directly, owing to the relatively wide spectral response of the photographic film.

The blur could be reduced by recording the hologram on a thicker material, but this would also reduce the apparent brightness of the image, and might also lead to processing difficulties and increased noise, even if it was a practical proposition.

However, if the hologram is recorded tilted (relative to the object, viewing, and reference source positions), the blurring can be dramatically reduced: minimum blur occurs when the reflection of the reference source in the hologram plane appears directly behind the object (corresponding to dispersion compensation in transmission holograms). This is illustrated in plate 1(c) which shows a hologram similar to that in plate 1(b), but recorded with a tilt of 20°; the large bright patch is the out-of-focus reflection of the illuminating source. This arrangement is clearly impractical for holographic displays, and so a compromise tilt must be chosen, taking into account the size of the hologram, the minimum distance of the observer, and the replay source position (which must be sufficiently high that the observer does not block it). A good arrangement for 30x40cm holograms is to have a reference angle of 45° with a backward tilt on the hologram of 15°, which allows the observer to approach the hologram to within 60mm of the hologram (along the z-axis) before having the source reflected into his eyes (closer if his eyes are above the z-axis). This compromise is illustrated by plate 1(d), which is clearly a significant improvement over the untilted hologram of plate 1(b).

The effect of tilting a hologram is illustrated quantitively in figure 10, which plots the calculated blur profile and wavelength of the dispersed image of object point (0,-100) for five values of tilt, as seen from a point on the z-axis (0,300), for holograms recorded with a reference at 30° to the z-axis. Note that the wavelength bandwidth of the blur is constant, which means that the brightness (total power diffracted) is also constant. These curves do not include an eye response factor.

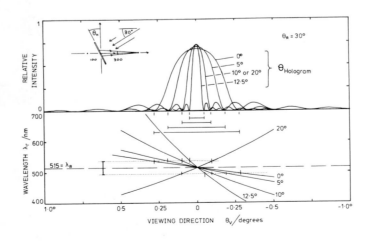

Fig. 10: The effect of tilt on the angular blur
in a reflection hologram

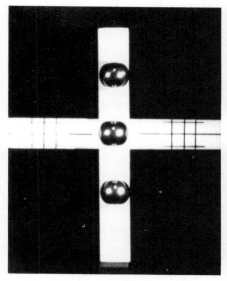

(a) Ideal replay source

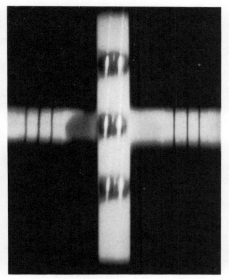

(b) white-light, no tilt

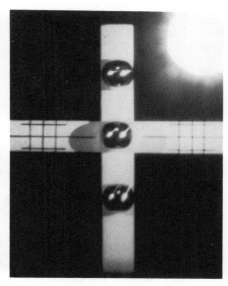

(c) white-light, 20° tilt

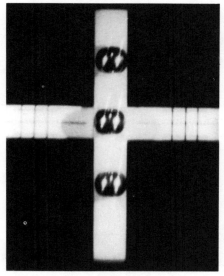

(d) white-light, 15° tilt

cm

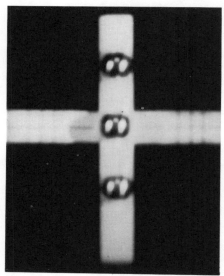

(e) 15° tilt; large source

Plate 1: Photographs of reflection holograms to show the effect of tilt and source size.

4. Conclusions

The various causes of blurring have been discussed. In particular, dispersion blurring has been modelled by combining ray-tracing with planar-grating coupled-wave equations; a result of the analysis being that dispersion blurring in reflection holograms may be reduced by recording the hologram with a tilt. It has further been shown that dispersion in transmission holograms may be made comparable with that in reflection holograms by using a sufficiently thick recording material.

Acknowledgements

The financial support of the Science and Engineering Research Council is gratefully acknowledged by the authors. We would also like to thank Pilkington Bros. for supplying the plates for our DCG experiments, and Alison for her patience in typing this manuscript.

References

1. A. A. Ward and L. Solymar, To be published. (J.Photo.Sci. 33, 1985, abstract only.)
2. C. B. Burkhardt, Bell Sys. Tech. J., 45, 1841-1844. 1966.
3. E. N. Leith, Scientific American 235, 80-95, (October 1976)
4. L. Solymar and D. J. Cooke, Academic Press, London, 1981, Chap. 3.
5. H. Kogelnik, Bell Sys. Tech. J., 48, 2909-2947, 1969.

Review of industrial applications of HOEs in display systems.

Emile J.P. SCHWEICHER

Centre de Recherches de l'Armée de Terre, TDLM/CT-TE,
Quartier Maj Housiau, Martelarenstraat 181, B-1801 Vilvoorde (Peutie). Belgium

Abstract

After a short review of diffractive optics, three display applications of HOEs are considered : helmet mounted displays, holographic night vision goggles and holographic head up displays. Possible future research fields are introduced.

Introduction

In recent years [9] holographic optical elements (HOEs) - which are also called diffractive optical elements (DOEs) - have found various applications. Important advantages are a low weight and a cheap manufacturing process. The most important imaging property of HOEs is that they can be tailored to any particular imaging geometry, independent of the orientation and curvature of the HOE substrate.

In contrast to classical optical lenses and mirrors based on refraction or reflection, DOEs have a grating-line structure and work by diffraction.

In what cases is it interesting to use DOEs ? A good rule [1] is that the more the imaging properties are required to deviate from those that would result from the laws of refraction and reflection, the stronger the dispersion, aberrations, and efficiency variations will be as the entering wave differs from the particular design assumptions. A "corollary" of this rule is that one should resort to the use of a HOE only when it is impossible to use conventional lenses and mirrors.

HOEs are now used in [9] laser beam scanners, head-up displays, fiber optic multiplexers and as lenses in optical systems. In this paper we are more particularly interested in the applications of HOEs in display systems.

Part I

Diffractive optics : a review.

1.1. Diffractive Optical Systems (DOEs) or Holographic Optical Elements (HOEs).

Basically there are two kinds of DOEs : holographic lenses and holographic mirrors although, in the literature, the word DOE generally stands for holographic mirror.

Holographic lenses are easily introduced by considering the recording set-up of fig. 1.a. where the reference wave is a coherent beam diverging from a point source R and the object wave is a coherent beam converging in O. As a matter of fact this recording process creates a transmission hologram since both recording beams are impinging from the same side upon the photosensitive plate P.

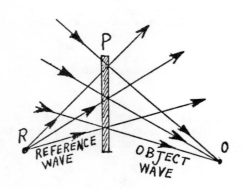

Fig. 1.a. Recording of a transmission hologram.

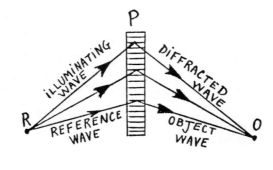

Fig. 1.b. Readout : converging holographic lens.

At readout (cfr fig. 1.b.) the hologram acts actually as a converging lens provided the diffraction efficiency is high enough to neglect the undiffracted or transmitted wave. Considering the overall orientation
of the fringes in a transmission hologram it is easily seen from fig. 1.b. that the "lens" working can be
understood by assuming   that each fringe surface acts as a mirror surface[1].

In the recording set-up of fig. 2.a., a reflection hologram is created by the interference of a converging coherent object beam and a diverging coherent reference beam impinging from opposite sides upon the
photosensitive plate P.

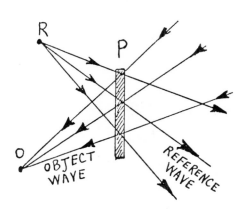

Fig. 2.a. Recording of a reflection hologram.

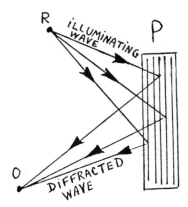

Fig. 2.b. Readout : holographic mirror.

At readout (cfr fig. 2.b.) this hologram acts actually as a concave mirror provided that the undiffracted
wave can be neglected; this last condition requires a fairly high value for the diffraction efficiency. Again
the "mirror" working can be understood by assuming that each fringe surface (see fig. 2.b.) acts as a mirror
surface.

The remainder of this paper is dealing only with holographic mirrors and their unique properties and applications. Consequently we shall be interested only by volume phase reflection holograms. The fringes -
which are also called Bragg layers - of such holograms are substantially oriented parallel to the substrate.

DOEs are subjected to the classical [9] aberrations : spherical aberration, field curvature, astigmatism,
coma, distortion and chromatic aberration. In some cases [14] the chromatic aberration is not an image aberration but the property on which the function of a HOE device is based. Most HOE-systems exhibit lack of rotation symmetry; therefore the aberrations (even the spherical aberration) have to be determined as a function of two coordinates.

The shape of the substrate influences the aberrations. It has already been stated in the introduction
that the more the imaging or the focusing properties - arising from the diffraction - are required to deviate
from those that would result from the laws of refraction and reflection, the stronger the dispersion and
aberrations will be. A "corollary" of this rule is that the shape of the fringes [11] should conform (i.e.
match) to the shape of the substrate which supports the recording photosensitive layer. If not the fringes
will be slanted and intersect the surface. These nonconformal fringes are to be avoided whenever possible
since they introduce chromatic aberration and can be detrimental in view of the finite bandwidth of the
phosphor screens used in display systems.

Many DOEs are not only required to reflect just like plane mirrors but they have also to exhibit focusing
properties (as seen, for instance, on fig. 2.b.). In such cases, the fringes will be curved; hence, a curved
substrate should then be prefered in order to minimize the aberrations, especially the chromatic aberration.

The validity of the rule of thumb stating that the fringes should conform to the substrate (in order to
reduce the chromatic aberration) can be easily shown by remembering that the "mirror" working of a DOE can be
understood (cfr fig. 2.b.) by assuming that each fringe surface acts as a mirror surface. For a spherical
curved DOE conformal fringes involve a DOE focal length equal to half of the radius of curvature of the substrate as usual for conventional spherical mirrors.

1.2. <u>Bragg's law and diffraction efficieny.</u>

In the case of a HOE designed to behave as a plane mirror, the fringes recorded will be essentially flat and parallel to the substrate. If we assume that the photosensitive recording material matches the refractive index of its substrate - as it is the case for dichromated gelatin (DCG) with a crown glass substrate (n = 1.5) - the HOE exhibits a grating-like structure which can be depicted by fig. 3 where d is the fringe spacing. Hence, Bragg's law shall be involved.

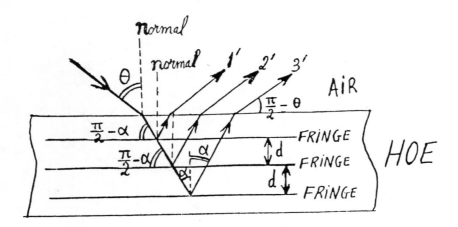

Fig. 3. Grating-like structure of a HOE : Bragg's law outline.

From Snell's law of refraction, the angle α is related to θ, the angle of incidence in air, by

$$\sin \theta = n \sin \alpha \tag{1}$$

where n is the refractive index of the recording photosensitive material. It is quite easy to show that the reflected rays 1', 2', 3', ... can only be in phase if d, the fringe spacing, is such that

$$2 d \cos \alpha = k\lambda/n \tag{2}$$

where $\begin{cases} \lambda \text{ is the free space wevelength} \\ k = 1, 2, 3, 4, \ldots \end{cases}$

Since $\cos \alpha = (1 - \sin^2\alpha)^{1/2}$ (3)

it can be deduced from (1), (2), (3) that

$$2d (n^2 - \sin^2\theta)^{1/2} = k\lambda \tag{4}$$

If the angle of incidence θ, the wavelength λ and the fringe spacing d do not fit in Bragg's law, the reflected rays 1', 2', 3', ... of fig. 3 become out of phase and interact destructively.

If the emulsion is sufficiently thick, the incident light intensity is reflected essentially into the first (i.e., k = 1) diffraction order, the higher diffraction orders (k = 2, 3, 4, ...) being substantially weak (less than 1%). For that reason, if we apply formula (4), we shall assume that the emulsion is sufficiently thick, so that k = 1.

Diffraction efficiency η is the ratio of the useful diffracted light flux to the total light flux used to illuminate the hologram at readout :

$$\eta = \frac{\text{diffracted flux}}{\text{illuminating flux}} \tag{5}$$

It should be interesting to establish theoretical expressions for the efficiency in order to emphasize the major influencing parameters.

Kogelnik [12] applied successfully the coupled wave theory to the problem of diffraction from volume holograms.

Kogelnik found that the achievement of the theoretical efficiency maximum requires two conditions simultaneously :

1° Bragg's law must be satisfied.

2° Unslanted fringe surfaces.

Pure phase volume reflection holograms are characterized by a high reflectivity over a narrow band of wavelengths, with the wavelength of peak reflectivity depending on the angle of incidence and the amount of expansion of the recording material between recording and use. The wavelength "Q" of the reflection hologram is approximately equal to the ratio of photosensitive emulsion thickness t to fringe spacing, i.e., the number N of fringes recorded in the thickness of the emulsion :

$$Q_\lambda \simeq \frac{t}{d} = N \tag{6}$$

The peak reflectivity of phase volume reflection holograms is given by the function

$$\eta_{max} = \tanh^2 \left(\frac{\pi \, \Delta n \, t}{\lambda_U \cos \theta_o} \right) \tag{7}$$

where : - λ_U is the free space wavelength during use.

- θ_o is the Bragg angle of incidence.

- Δn is the refractive index modulation.

1.3. Gelatin DOEs - Dichromated gelatin (DCG) [13] [15].

HOEs are made using dichromated gelatin (DCG), which is presently the only material capable of providing the necessary qualities. This situation could change dramatically in the future because new recording materials such as photopolymers are being studied to reduce exposure time and processing complexity as well as to increase environmental stability.

Gelatin is a fibrous protein collagen from animal skin and bones. Although [13] a gelatin film is not intrinsically sensitive to light, it is nevertheless possible, through chemical sensitization, to induce changes in the gelatin itself corresponding to an incident light pattern, allowing the recording of very high efficiency volume phase holograms.

Different sensitization chemical products (i.e. products rendering the gelatin photosensitive) can be used. Ammonium dichromate $(NH_4)_2 Cr_2 O_7$ is a sensitization material which seems to be the best trade-off between several requirements; consequently, gelatin impregnated with ammonium dichromate has become a standard holographic recording material. It is only recently [13] that the use of silver halide photographic emulsions to produce gelatin holograms, pioneered several years ago, has received further attention.

The photosensitive properties of dichromated gelatin (DCG) and other chromated and dichromated organic substances have been known for about 150 years. It has been [13] claimed from time to time that the properties of DCG as a volume holographic recording material are close to ideal. The DCG hologram formed during normal exposures to laser light is of very low efficiency, so the material has the advantages of latent image type operation. It is almost grainless and exhibits very high spatial resolution - more than 5000 mm^{-1} - and low scattering at readout, so that high signal-to-noise ratios are possible. In addition, the recorded holograms are highly stable, because [15] DCG is unaffected by moisture, exposure to ultraviolet light and temperatures up to 90°C, provided DCG is sealed between two layers of glass to avoid contact with moisture.

The most significant disadvantage of DCG is its comparatively low sensitivity (what requires long exposure times) which, depending upon the source of the gelatin, is a factor of around 100 down on fine grain photographic emulsions such as Agfa 8E56HD or Kodak 649F. The recording of a DOE in a DCG film is usually carried out at 488 nm or 514.5 nm (both being spectral lines of the Ar laser), for which the full thickness of a 15 μm (which seems to be a standard thickness for a DCG recording film) emulsion can be exposed.

The mechanism of the photochemical process which occurs when the DCG film is exposed to light is not wholly understood. It is generally [13] accepted, however, that absorption of light is by the Cr^{6+} ion, and that reduction occurs to Cr^{3+} ions, as a result of a reaction with the gelatin which causes cross-linking of the gelatin molecules, thereby inducing local hardening (proportional to the local light intensity) in the bulk of the gelatin layer.

The preceding cross-linking could be represented as follows :

The local hardening implies a spatial variation of the refractive index (i.e., a refractive index modulation Δn). Hence a volume phase hologram is obtained.

After the exposure to the laser light during the recording phase of the HOE, the hologram has to undergo a development procedure; the purpose of this development is to amplify (this is necessary since it has already been claimed that the hologram formed during normal exposures to laser light is of very low efficiency) the refractive index modulation Δn - thereby increasing (cfr formula 7) highly the efficiency - and to fix it definitely.

The development consists of an initial washing in water - to desensitive the plate by removing all remaining Cr^{6+} ions - followed by a treatment with isopropanol; finally the development is completed by a fast drying in a hot air flow (150°C) followed by a slow drying (several hours) in free atmosphere.

During the washing in water, the DCG layer undergoes an enormous swelling (about a factor 20). Afterwards (during the treatment with isopropanol), the alcohol causes rapid dehydration and shrinkage of the gelatin. The development procedure is in fact found [13] to be reversible so that immersion of the processed hologram in water reduces the efficiency once more to a very low value and processing can be repeated at least a few cycles. Despite the considerable changes in thickness which the DCG film undergoes during processing, some degree of control is possible over the thickness of the final hologram, and therefore the peak reconstruction (i.e., readout) wavelength λ_{max} (see para 1.4.).

Slight loss of efficiency with time can be expected under any conditions, but [13] steady deterioration has been observed at 50% humidity and rapid destruction at 70%, so that sealing is necessary for protection. Reprocessing will, however, restore the efficiency.

Sealing is done normally by covering the gelatin with a glass shell which is tighten to the gelatin by means of an appropriate adhesive. The purpose of sealing is manifold : protect, preserve efficiency, stop interaction with atmosphere, thereby freezing the evolution in time of the peak reconstruction wavelength λ_{max} (which will be defined in the next paragraph).

The temperature is the major degrading factor of a DCG hologram. This has to be taken into account for storage conditions. For instance, a holographic HUD has been destroyed after staying 5 hours at a temperature above 80°C.

The average refractive index of DCG after recording of the HOE is 1.55 which is nearly the value of the refractive index before exposure to laserlight. This value matches almost 1.523 which is the value of the refractive index of the crown glass substrate.

The manufacturing process [15] of a HOE requires the closely controlled environment of a specially designed clean room facility. Not only must the atmosphere be dust-free but the specified temperature and humidity levels must be tightly maintained.

Cleanliness is important at all stages but especially in the film preparation, to avoid particles becoming trapped in the gelatin. Relative humidity control is necessary to ensure reproducibility of tuning and efficiency.

Vibration isolation [15] is also important for the laser exposure during which movements of as little as one tenth of the wavelength of light can be significant. Kaiser Electronics - probably the world's largest HUD supplier - has [6] a diffraction-optics subsidiary which is located in Ann Harbor, Michigan, rather than in the company's seismically unstable home territoy of San Jose, California.

1.4. Wavelength (or spectral) selectivity of the HOEs.

Since volume holograms exhibit a grating-like structure, it was stated (after Kogelnik [12]) in paragraph 1.2. that the achievement of a maximum diffraction efficiency requires 2 conditions :
1° Unslanted fringes.
2° Bragg's law should be satisfied.

For a fixed angle of incidence θ_o, it is seen from (4) that only one wavelength λ_{max} fits into Bragg's law.   Consequently the plots of the reflectance R and of the transmittance T as a function of wavelength should be those of fig. 4, exhibiting either a maximum (for R) or a minimum (for T) at the peak wavelength λ_{max} and a waveband $\Delta\lambda$ which is clearly defined on the plot of R as being the width of the peak at 50% reflectance although it is more often measured at 50% transmittance, there being [11] very little difference and the latter being more easily measurable.

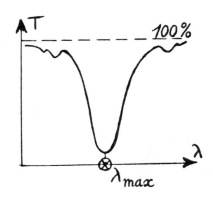

Fig. 4. Reflectance and transmittance versus wavelength for a given angle of incidence.

Figure 4 outlines the wavelength selectivity (also called spectral selectivity) of HOEs, i.e. their unique ability to provide a high degree of reflection in a clearly defined waveband (also called spectral bandwidth) $\Delta\lambda$, coupled with almost complete transparency outside it.

In the case of unslanted fringes, R_{max}, the maximum reflectance of fig. 4, is nothing else but η_{max} given by equation 7. Hence, for underslanted fringes :

$$R_{max} = \tanh^2 \left(\frac{\pi.\Delta n.t}{\lambda_{max} \cos \theta_o}\right) \qquad (8)$$

where θ_o is the Bragg angle of incidence corresponding to λ_{max}.

As a matter of fact, λ_{max}, the peak reconstruction wavelength, would be equal to λ_R, the recording wavelength, if t, the thickness of the photosensitive layer, would not be altered during the development procedure. Generally this is not true. In paragraph 1.3. it was stated that DCG is presently the most widely used recording material. It has also been seen that the development procedure of a DCG recorded DOE implies a swelling followed by a shrinkage. A swelling implies an increase of the fringe spacing d, while a shrinkage provokes a decrease of d. Consequently, it follows from Bragg's law (4) that λ_{max}, the peak reconstruction wavelength, is generally not equal to the wavelength λ_R which is often one of the following spectral lines of the Ar laser : 488 nm or, more frequently, 514.5 nm.

The final step of the development procedure of DCG consists of a slow drying in free atmosphere. During this step, the shrinkage goes on - thereby decreasing λ_{max} - until it is stopped by the sealing. Consequently, λ_{max}, the peak readout wavelength, can be almost tuned to any value not too far from λ_R.

Since the wavelength "Q" is classicaly defined as (cfr fig. 4)

$$Q_\lambda = \lambda_{max}/\Delta\lambda \qquad (9)$$

it follows from (6) that

$$\Delta\lambda \simeq \lambda_{max}/N \qquad (10)$$

where N is the number of fringes recorded in the thickness t of the photosensitive layer.

If a flat HOE has been designed to behave as a plane mirror reflecting a diverging beam issued from a point source, the fringes recorded will be essentially flat and parallel but will vary in spacing over the exposed area according to Bragg's law (4) because the angle of incidence θ is varying over the exposed area. This effect can be illustrated by the wavelength selectivity curves (cfr fig. 6) of a flat beam splitting HOE designed (cfr fig. 5) to reflect an incident diverging beam at area A, and to transmit a collimated beam at area B. The curves of fig. 6 have been recorded with the same diverging beam which is impinging under the same incidence either on area A or area B.

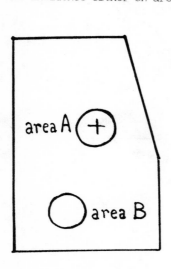

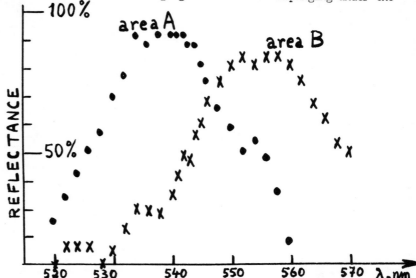

Fig. 5. Beam splitter reflecting at area A and transmitting at area B.

Fig. 6. Wavelength selectivity of the beam splitter of fig. 5.

1.5. Angular selectivity of the HOEs.

For a fixed wavelength λ_o, it is seen from (4) that only one angle of incidence θ_{max} fits into Bragg's law. Consequently, a HOE features also an angular selectivity, i.e. a unique ability to provide a high degree of reflection in an angular bandwith $\Delta\theta$ located around θ_{max}, coupled with almost complete transparency outside it.

Woodcock [11] has published a nice example of the usefulness of angular selectivity : fig. 8 gives the plot of the reflectance versus the angle of incidence for the beam splitting HOE of the quasi-axial combiner configuration depicted by fig. 7.

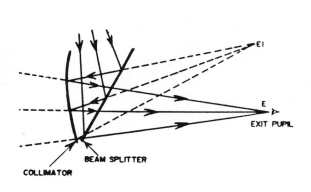

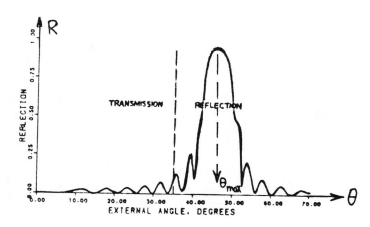

Fig. 7. A quasi-axial combiner configuration[11].

Fig. 8. Angular selectivity of the beam splitter of fig. 7 (fixed wavelength)[11].

It is easy to show that the angular selectivity is in close relationship with the wavelength selectivity. From Bragg's law (4) it can be deduced that the peak reflection wavelength λ_{max} versus the angle of incidence θ is given by

$$\lambda_{max} = \lambda_o \left(1 - \frac{\sin^2 \theta}{n^2}\right)^{1/2} \tag{11}$$

where λ_o is the tuning wavelength at normal incidence.

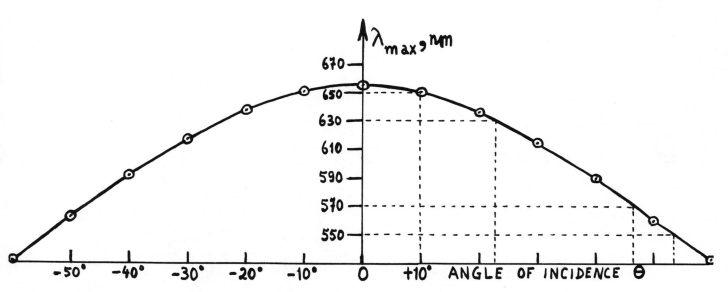

Fig. 9. The change of peak wavelength with angle of incidence.

It is obvious that the function (11) is even as can be seen on the experimental record of fig. 9 which has been taken on a flat HOE by means of transmittance measurements using a collimated beam.

Figure 9 shows the relation between angular and spectral bandwidths : for angles close to normal incidence the angular bandwidth of a given HOE is appreciably greater than for angles of around 45°. This effect can be seen in fig. 10 which has been computed by Woodcock [11] and shows the reflectance against angle of incidence for a particular hologram (hence, figure 10 characterizes the angular selectivity). The different peaks of fig. 10 were obtained by using different reconstruction wavelengths.

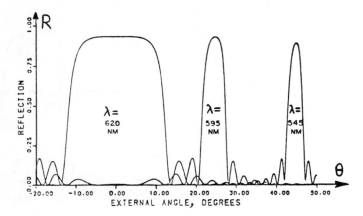

Fig. 10. The reflection efficiency characteristics for peaks at different angles and wavelengths [11].

From fig. 10 it can be seen that the peak reflectance R_{max} is decreasing when the angle of incidence increases. It is possible to explain that by a polarization effect which can be clearly seen on the experimental record of fig. 11 which has been taken from a flat HOE designed to behave as a plane mirror for the maximum eye sensitivity wavelength at an angle of incidence close to the Brewster angle of DCG and substrate.

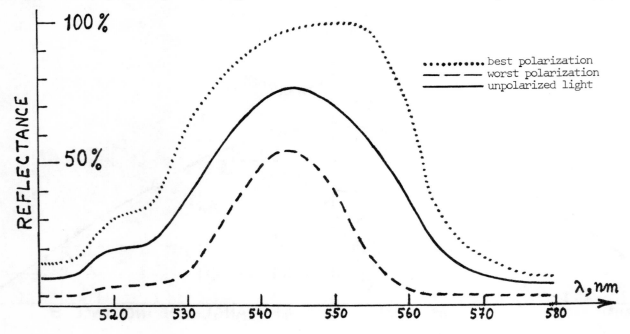

Fig. 11. Polarization effect close to the Brewster angle.

Other experiments have shown that the discrepancy between both linear polarizations decreases when the angle of incidence decreases.
Remark :
Many DOEs are characterized by a peak reconstruction wavelength (cfr fig. 4) λ_{max} = 543 nm which is the central wavelength of the phosphor screens P20, P43 and P53 which are so useful in military applications. As

these DOEs are acting [8] as highly efficient reflectors over narrow spectral bandwidths surrounding 543 nm, the corresponding part of the outside world spectrum will be "lost" as it is transmitted through the DOE; so there will be some slight pink coloration on the outside scene.

Part II

Applications of HOEs in display systems.

2.1. Generalities.

A good quality HOE will reflect about 90% of the light over a narrow ($\Delta\lambda$ of fig. 4 is of the order of 15 nm for a thickness t = 15 μm) spectral region whilst efficiently transmitting other wavelengths. Since most display systems are using phosphor screens it is necessary that the light generated by those screens lies in the same narrow waveband in order to be efficiently reflected. Consequently the standard P20 phosphor screen - which matches so well the eye sensitivity - cannot be used since its spectrum occupies a waveband of 200 nm located around 535 nm. For applications of HOEs in display systems, it is mandatory to resort to special narrow band phosphor screens such as P43 and P53, both being characterized by a central wavelength of 543 nm and, unfortunately, by a photometric efficiency (in lm/W) lower than that of the P20 screen.

2.2. Helmet mounted display.

A helmet mounted display (for aircraft or helicopter pilots) is an optical system that images [1] a CRT (cathode ray tube) surface to infinity, without obstructing the wearer's view. A "reflection" HOE sandwiched in the helmet visor and conforming to the shape of the visor directs light from a conventional optical system on the side of the helmet into the wearer's eye. To accomplish this, the chief ray (in Ref 1) is reflected from an angle of incidence of 47° into (cfr fig. 12) an angle of 13° on the same side of the normal to the surface. Optical power in the HOE images the system pupil into the eye pupil of the wearer, thus providing a bright image. This geometry could not have been achieved with conventional optics.

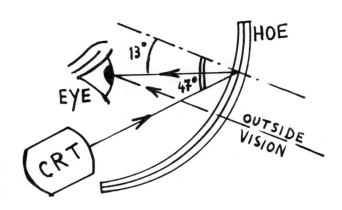

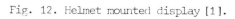

Fig. 12. Helmet mounted display [1].

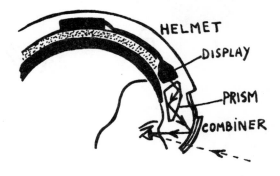

Fig. 12. bis. Cutaway drawing of the Marconi helmet mounted display. A moving display is generated and focusses ad infinity [17].

In France [10] Thomson - CSF is actively investigating helmet-mounted sights. In the USA [16] Honeywell-Austin is working on a helmet sight for the future ATF (Advanced Tactical Fighter) and Hughes is developing a helmet with a head-up visor display, which is part of a new helicopter night vision system developed to improve a pilot's vision on low level missions at night, in adverse weather or in hazy and smoky conditions : in flight, a forward-looking infrared (FLIR) image, which resembles a black and white TV picture, is projected onto the helmet visor so the pilot may see the world outside the cockpit.

Recently it was announced [5] that a new helmet-mounted cockpit display is under development by the Air Force Aerospace Medical Research Laboratory (AFAMRL) at Wright-Patterson AFB, Ohio. The helmet prototype developed at AFAMRL employs two circular, 1-in.-diameter CRTs - one for each eye. A complex optical system linked to each CRT bends, magnifies, and collimates the image, projecting it into the pilot's eye. Each eye sees a 60°-vertical-by-80°-horizontal field of view. One change for the flight model calls for a holographic see-through visor, so that in daylight the pilot can view the real world as well as a simulated scene. To further reduce the helmet weight, AFAMRL engineers are planning to use smaller CRTs, probably about 0.8 in. in diameter. Thomas Electronics Inc. supplied the 1-in. CRTs and is working on smaller versions. The Air Force has also contracted with Hughes Aircraft Co. and AT & T laboratories to develop smaller CRTs.

2.3. Holographic night vision goggles.

This optical system - which is depicted in fig. 13 - uses a HOE in conjunction with a relay lens assembly - which consists of additional, conventional optical systems - to image the exit phosphor screen of an I^2T (Image Intensifier Tube) to infinity (collimation); hence, the wearer's eye doesn't have to accomodate; this prevents eye fatigue.

Since the goggles have to be portable, the I^2T shall be a MCP (Micro-Channel Plate) second or third generation tube. The peak reflectivity wavelength λ_{max} of the HOE (cfr fig. 8) must be tuned to 543 nm, which is the central wavelength of the "monochromatic" phosphor screen. Consequently the HOE shall exhibit a high reflectivity in a narrow waveband around 543 nm, coupled with almost complete transparency outside it; hence, these goggles exhibit a see-through capability which can be very useful in twilight conditions.

But the main advantage of the see-through capability shows up when an intense lighting appears suddenly on the battlefield; in that case the intensified image loses its contrasts (this phenomenon is due to the self-saturating characteristics of the microchannels inside the I^2T) and, finally, the intensified image gets smeared (there is no blooming danger with a second or third generation I^2T). In that case, the wearer of conventional night vision goggles would be obliged to take them off. Thanks to the see-through capability, the wearer of holographic night vision goggles may keep his goggles since a direct view of the outside world (in ambient light) will be granted to him.

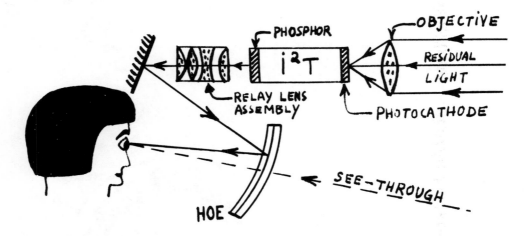

Fig. 13. Holographic night vision goggles (see-through capability).

In the UK, Pilkington seems to have already realized some prototypes, of holographic night vision goggles. In the USA, some years ago, prototypes of the Hughes HOT (holographic on tube) goggles have been tested by the Army. In Belgium, the Army evaluated in 1985 (laboratory and field trials) prototypes of HNV goggles developed by OIP.
Remark : As a matter of fact, the see-through capability would also exist if one replaces the HOE of fig. 13 by a conventional beam-splitter (i.e. a half reflecting mirror). A conventional beam-splitter exhibits a reflectance of about 50% almost independently of the wavelength whereas a HOE exhibits a much higher reflectance in a narrow waveband which corresponds precisely with the narrow spectral emission of the I^2T phosphor screen. Consequently, holographic night vision goggles are less detectable by the enemy (considering the green phosphor exiting light) and are characterized by a high brightness of the intensified image as seen by the wearer.

2.4. Head Up Display (HUD). [8][6][10][15].

Most of the recent Western multi-role aircrafts (Mirage 2000, F-16, F-15, F/A-18, A-7 Corsair) are one-man designs, leaving the F-14 and the Tornado as the only recent air combat types with a two-man crew.

The new Western multi-mission types on the horizon are [10] all set for one-man operation : the EFA European Fighter Aircraft, Israel's LAVI, Sweden's JAS-39 GRIPEN and the Swiss PIRANHA.

The displays - i.e. head-down displays, head-up displays, helmet mounted displays - are the key [10] to the one-man cockpit.

Aircraft Head Up Display (HUD) systems provide the pilot with essential flight, navigation, and in the case of military aircraft, weapon aiming information. Fig. 14 shows a conventional HUD comprising the CRT display, the relay lens assembly and a flat combiner.

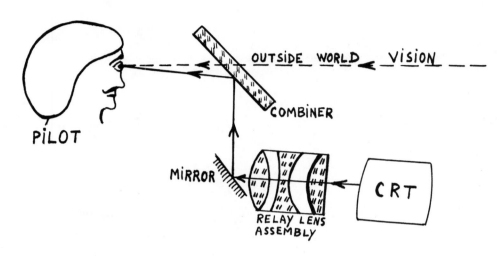

Fig. 14. Conventional HUD.

Information generated on a high resolution CRT is collimated [15] by the relay lens assembly so as to produce an image at infinity which is seen by the pilot after reflection in a partially reflecting plate known as the combiner. The pilot thereby sees the display superimposed on his view of the outside world. The pilot is thus able to fly the aircraft "head up" thereby reducing workload and enhancing his weapon aiming capability. As the display will sometimes be used for weapon aiming, the collimating lens must be very high quality so that the accuracy of the overlay on the real world is maintained over a range of eye positions and over the required field of view. The lens must also be fast (F number approaching 1). Apart from the CRT itself, the other factor which controls the display brightness is the reflectivity of the combiner plate. The combiner cuts down the light coming in from the outside world, darkening the field of view and in turn increasing the difficulty of detecting surface targets, especially in bad weather.

Since the combiner must be as transparent as possible to allow the pilot [15] to see the outside world in conditions of poor visibility, and yet behave as a mirror for the CRT display, a compromise is necessary. It is generally accepted that the combiner must pass 72% of the light from outside. This implies that it can reflect at most 28% of the available light from the display using conventional semi-reflecting coatings and giving a maximum display luminance of [8] around 5000 Nit. The luminance and display contrast requirements are only achieved with [8] the CRT producing maximum luminance (typically 35,000 Nit), a level which will reduce its life.

The HUD was initially a purely sighting device. It now is required [15] to display a wide range of information including Forward Looking Infra-Red (FLIR) imagery for low-altitude night-interdiction missions - i.e. low-altitude navigation and target acquisition at night - on pre-planned targets. Pilots flying at 600 knots or so "on the deck" need to be able to "see" the countryside not just ahead but around them as well. This has led to a continual demand for increased sophistication of the HUDs.

Particular areas [15] requiring improvement are the display brightness and the (instantaneous) FOV (field of view). For daytime flying at high altitude a very high brightness is necessary if the display is to be visible against a background of sunlit clouds, for instance. Night flying, on the other hand, may demand a FLIR Raster Display, for which a wide FOV is required, superimposed on the pilot's view of the world outside. While a 20° FOV can be used for night attack, a 30° FOV immeasurably improves effectiveness and piloting ease.

Holography can contribute to both these areas. By contrast with conventional HUD's, holographic HUD's can virtually double the FOV and achieve [15] with a P43 phosphor a display reflectivity of 58% while the outside world transmission remains at 72%. Thanks to this improvement of display reflectivity, the CRT can be run at lower luminance - a peak display luminance [8] of around 8500 Nit may be achieved - i.e. the CRT is underrun under normal conditions thereby prolonging its life. Compared [14] with conventional, mirrored glass displays, the holographic HUD has a wider FOV, is more transparent, has brighter symbology and reduces glare and sunballs.

2.5. Holographic HUD or DHUD. [15][6][11].

A DHUD (Diffractive optics HUD) is "simply" a HUD where the combiner is a HOE having a spectral response which is matched [8] to the CRT P43 (or P53) phosphor. Replacing the flat conventional combiner of fig. 14 by a "well tuned" flat HOE affects [15] only the display luminance. In order to improve the FOV, the optical layout must be rearranged.

A considerable advantage [15] can be gained by incorporating the collimator into the combiner as has be done [6] for many years in the design of astronomical telescopes and, more recently, in the design of long-focus camera lenses, by the use of light curved mirrors to replace lenses.

A single curved HOE can satisfy [15] both functions (collimator and combiner) or a combination of HOEs may be used. Figure 15 shows the case for a single HOE. The lens in this system does not collimate the light from the CRT but re-focusses it to form an intermediate image in the focal plane of the curved HOE. The curved HOE behaves as a concave mirror and by collimating the light makes the image appear to be at infinity. DHUDS of this type (fig. 15) have been developed by Hughes, Kaiser and Thomson-CSF[6][10].

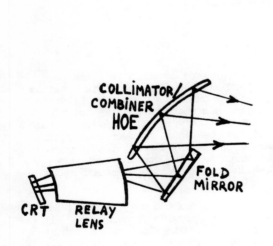

Fig. 15. DHUD with single curved HOE [15].

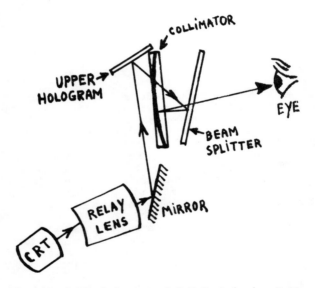

Fig. 16. Optical layout of G.E.C. Avionics F-16 LANTIRN DHUD [8].

Field of view improvement [15] is achieved in two ways. First, the HOE can be wider than was feasible with the lens collimator, and second, it can be nearer to the pilot's eyes.

A further example (see fig. 16) is the G.E.C. Avionics F-16 LANTIRN (Low Altitude Navigation and Targeting by Infra-Red at Night) DHUD with optics manufactured by Pilkington [8][11][15]. In this case a combination of 3 HOEs (upper hologram, collimator, beam splitter) is used but the principle is just the same. Figure 17 shows the degree of improvement in FOV which can be obtained in this way, comparing as it does the conventional F-16 C/D HUD with the LANTIRN DHUD for the same aircraft.

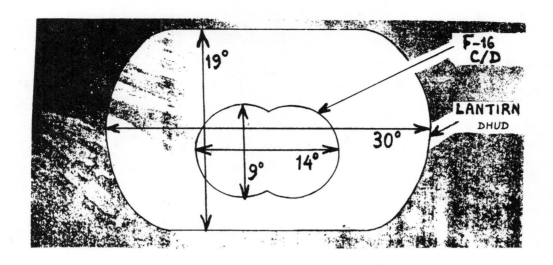

Fig. 17. FOV comparison between F-16 C/D (small area) and F-16 LANTIRN (large area) [15][8].

The LANTIRN DHUD is an attractive system combining spectral and angular selectivities. The curved collimating HOE (see fig. 16) must necessarily collimate but is also required to transmit a view of the outside world. The beam splitter HOE must perform three roles :
(1) transmit a clear view of the outside world.
(2) efficiently reflect the display onto the collimator.
(3) efficiently transmit the collimated display to the pilot.

Thanks to the reflectance curve of fig. 19 the beam splitter HOE is able to perform these three tasks simultaneously. Compared to the combiner configuration of fig. 7, Woodcock [11] says that the combiner (see fig. 18)

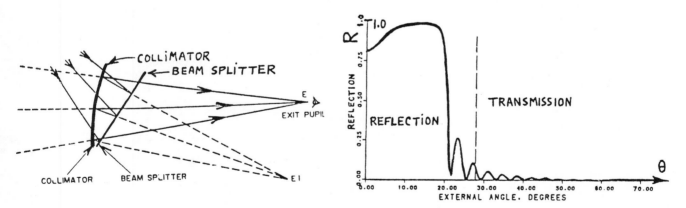

Fig. 18. An improved quasi-axial combiner configuration [11].

Fig. 19. Reflection characteristic of the beam splitter element in figure 18 [11].

of the LANTIRN DHUD is an improved configuration because :
(1) the combiner of fig. 7 would have a problem of sun reflection due to the uptilt of the collimator; the LAN-TIRN configuration (fig. 18) avoids this by tilting the collimator downwards.
(2) in fig. 8 the angles requiring transmission are closer to normal incidence than the reflection peak. In fig. 19 the reverse is true with the reflection peak occupying the smaller angles. This is a further advantage for the LANTIRN DHUD since the angular bandwidth requirement is more easily met as was seen during the discussion about angular selectivity (cfr fig.10).

But the combiner configuration of the LANTIRN DHUD (fig. 18) has probably another advantage with respect to the configuration of fig. 7 : due to the polarization effect illustrated by fig. 11, the maximum reflectance of the beam splitter of fig. 7 is necessarily lower than that of the beam splitter of fig. 18 which is working closer to normal incidence.

2.6. Future research fields in diffractive optics [6].

Whatever the fortunes of the present generation of DHUDs, the potential of diffraction optics is considered high in all quarters. Colour DHUDs, hitherto impratical, can be made with three superimposed holograms, each reflecting one primary colour. "It is easy to make multiple holograms" muses one engineer. "The problem is making the ones we want"[6]. However, the feeling is that the user community is becoming accustomed to the much faster and more positive visual cues which are possible with colour displays, and that the demand for colour DHUDs will be there if they can be manufactured at reasonable cost.

In the longer term, some designers are looking at ways to remove conventional refraction (i.e. the lenses used in the recording setups) and reflection from the manufacturing process; instead of splitting and focusing the recording laser beam by mirrors and lenses, the hologram could be exposed point by point, using a computer-controlled laser. In this way, any optical property which can be defined by computer can be produced, and, in theory, the entire optical system of a DHUD could be reduced to two holograms and the CRT. Research into such devices, called COHOEs (Computer-Originated Holographic Optical Elements) is under way. While current efforts are largely directed towards the development of the first-generation systems (the DHUDs explained in paragraph 2.5.) now on order, the practical application of diffraction optics in aerospace has only begun.

In all cases, future research will probably involve :
- improvement of diffraction efficiency.
- reduction of aberrations.
- reproducibility in the manufacturing process of HOEs.
- improvement of environmental characteristics.
- duplication of a master hologram for series production.
- looking for other photosensitive recording materials than DCG, e.g. photopolymers.

Acknowledgements.

The author wishes to express his sincere thanks to prof. Dr. Lagasse and prof. Keil for their support and discussions and to Mrs Monique Troch for typing the manuscript.

References.

1. D.H. CLOSE "Optical recorded holographic optical elements"; pp 573-585 in "Handbook of optical holography" edited by H.J. CAUFIELD, Academic Press, 1979.
2. M. FRANÇON "Holographie", Masson, Paris, 1969.
3. J. KEIL "Holographie", Travaux pratiques de physique, Facultés Universitaires Notre-Dame de la Paix, Namur, 1982.
4. Science/Scope, p. 56, Military Technology, Vol. 8, Issue 9, 1984.
5. W.R. IVERSEN "Helmet gives graphic pictures", p. 34, Electronics Week, April 1, 1985.
6. B. SWEETMAN "US manufacturers move on advanced HUDs", pp 34-37, Special Electronics N° 2/1984, Supplement to Vol. 17-9, International Defense Review, 1984.
7. A. THEVENON "Aberrations of holographic gratings", pp 308-315, SPIE Proc. Vol. 399, April 19-22, 1983, Geneva, Switzerland.
8. C.H. VALLANCE "The approach to optical system designs for aircraft head up displays", pp 15-25, SPIE Proc. Vol. 399, April 19-22, 1983, Geneva, Switzerland.
9. J. VAN ROEY & W. DE WILDE "Ray tracing program for holographic optical elements", pp 316-322, SPIE Proc. Vol 399, April 19-22, 1983, Geneva, Switzerland.
10. M. WILSON "Displays, key to one-man cockpit", pp 26-33, Special Electronics N° 2/1984, Supplement to Vol 17-9, International Defense Review, 1984.
11. B.H. WOODCOCK "Volume phase holograms and their application to avionic displays", pp 333-338, SPIE Proc. 399, April 19-22, 1983, Geneva, Switzerland.
12. H. KOGELNIK, Bell Syst. Tech. Journal, Vol 48, p 2909 (1969).
13. L. SOLYMAR & D.J. COOKE "Volume holography and volume gratings", pp 278-286, Academic Press, 1981.
14. J.L. HORNER & J.E. LUDMAN "Single Holographic Element Wavelength Demultiplexer", Appl. Optics, Vol 20, N° 10, pp 1845-1847, 1981.
15. B.H. WOODCOCK & A.J. KIRKHAM "Holographic applications in avionics HUDs", pp 94-97, MILTECH 6/85.
16. B. SWEETMAN "The cockpit of the US ATF", International Defense Review, pp 687-689, 5/1985.
17. D.J. WALKER "Helmet mounted systems", pp 28-31, MILTECH 9/83.

SOME RESEARCH TOWARD THE DEVELOPMENT OF A HOLOGRAM LASER BEAM CORRECTOR—COLLIMATOR FOR USE IN A SATELLITE DATA LINK

C. Gilbreath-Frandsen
William H. Carter
Naval Research Laboratory
Washington, D.C. 20375
and
J. W. Wagner
Johns Hopkins University
Department of Materials Science and Engineering
Baltimore, MD 21218

ABSTRACT

Some initial research results are reported toward developing holographic optical elements for use as beam corrector-collimators for diode laser arrays in an inter-satellite data link. Holograms have been made in 649F emulsions with 633 nm radiation from a He-Ne laser under conditions which simulate a hologram made in an IR-sensitive emulsion with a diode laser. Such holograms have been copied into dichromated gelatin emulsions with 488 nm radiation from an Ar+ laser. The copies have shown up to 94% efficiency when reconstructed as optical elements at 633 nm. Some difficulties in obtaining efficient holograms that do not introduce significant wavefront aberrations are discussed and possible solutions described.

I. INTRODUCTION

We are studying the use of holograms as optical elements to correct aberrated wavefronts from diode lasers and coherent diode laser arrays in order to produce well-collimated beams suitable for use in free space optical communications between satellites. Laser diodes and diode arrays are uniquely suited to spacecraft communica-tions because of their small size and mass. However, they do present some problems. Single diode lasers produce diverging cones of light that are highly astigmatic, as shown in Fig. 1. These devices also lack the power needed for a communications system. Coherent diode arrays have sufficient power but produce rapidly diverging cones of light with highly irregular wavefronts. Thus, the radiation from such a device must be transformed by an optical system which corrects the aberrated wavefront, collimates the beam, and then directs it toward the receiver.

Conventional optical systems like that shown in Fig. 2 are presently used to transform the beams from single diode lasers. Such systems include many lenses and an anamorphic prism pair to correct the astigmatism. They are quite massive for satellite use and the lasers produce inadequate light. No really suitable optical system is available to efficiently transform the beam from a diode laser array because of the complexity of the wavefront. Thus, the increased power available from these arrays is not fully available.

It would be a great advantage if holograms could be used in place of conventional optics to transform these

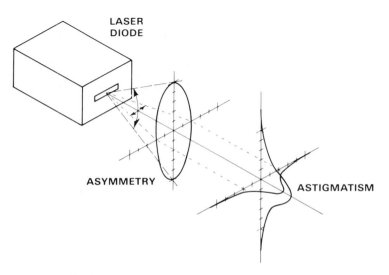

Fig. 1 — Aberrated Output Beam from a Laser Diode.

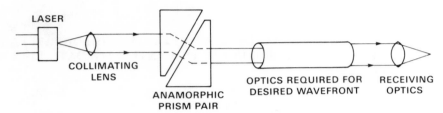

Fig. 2 — Conventional Optical System for Correcting the Output from a Laser Diode.

laser beams. Holograms are thin, low in mass, and appear to be rugged. A single hologram can perform the same operations as a complex optical system. Furthermore, a hologram can perform operations which cannot be performed by conventional optical systems. It appears possible that they can be used to efficiently correct the complicated wavefront aberrations in a beam from a diode laser array. The application of holograms as beam transformers in satellite communications links was suggested previously by Carter and Caulfield (Ref. 1), and some difficulties and possible solutions were described.

II. APPROACH

The most straightforward approach to obtaining such a hologram would be to expose a holographic emulsion to the interference pattern formed between the aberrated light cone directly from the diode laser or laser diode array and a replica of a good communications beam obtained by beam splitting, spatially filtering, and collimating the light from the same source. After developing, the hologram would serve as an optical system to transform the light cone from the source into the communications beam as shown in Fig. 3. The obvious difficulty with this approach is the unavailability of high-resolution, IR-sensitive, photographic emulsions capable of producing efficient holograms. The question, then, is what can we do with the materials available.

There are several possibilities. The one we have chosen to explore in our work thus far is a two-step process involving a master hologram made with a diode laser in an IR- sensitive material which does not produce efficient holograms, and a second, working hologram copied from the master into dichromated gelatin with 488 nm from an Ar+ laser to obtain an efficient hologram (Refs. 1 and 2).

The main advantage of this approach is that the master hologram is made directly with the aberrated wavefront from the actual diode laser. Thus, it may accurately transform the light from the laser into a communications beam even though the laser produces light with a very complicated wavefront. No wavefront simulations or complicated optical designs are required. A second advantage is that the final hologram made in dichromated gelatin can be made to be very efficient so that almost all of the light from the laser diode is transformed into the "communications" beam.

A disadvantage is that if the working hologram is replicated from the master by a direct contact printing process, the working hologram is limited by the low resolution of the master hologram. For the Kodak spectroscopic IVN emulsion which we are using, the maximum resolution is about 200 to 250 lp/mm. This low resolution limits the grating period in the holograms to about 4 microns and the Bragg angle to no more than 5.8 degrees.

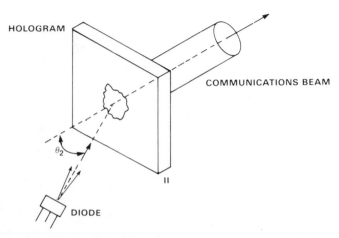

Fig. 3 — Holographic Optical System to Correct and Collimate a Diode Laser Beam.

This presents a serious limitation in systems design. Also, if the dichromated gelatin hologram is to be efficient, it must satisfy a mathematical condition that the emulsion be thick or that the grating spacing be small (Ref. 3). For typical diode wavelengths relevant to this application (750 nm to 900 nm), using IVN emulsion, the thickness must be as much as 127 microns for holograms with grating periods on the order of 4 microns. Thicknesses of this magnitude are problematic, as it has been found that dichromated gelatin emulsions of thicknesses greater than 50 microns require special techniques which are still experimental (Ref. 4). If the working hologram is a copy made through holographic reconstruction of the master, aberrations will be introduced due to the wavelength shift. However, a theoretical study has been made which indicates that through proper construction and reconstruction geometries, these aberrations will be automatically corrected when the working hologram is reconstructed with the same Infrared wavelength used to make the master hologram (Ref. 2).

In this paper, we will present a heuristic argument to explain the physical basis of the thick emulsion/small grating spacing condition for hologram efficiency, describe a proof-of-concept experiment for producing very efficient holographic optical elements using the two-step method described above, and describe some preliminary results employing a stable single-mode diode to make the master hologram using spectroscopic IVN emulsion.

III. THEORY

One of the most difficult problems in making a hologram that is useful as an optical element is making a hologram that is efficient such that it diffracts almost all of the incident light into the required beam. Diffraction of light from grating structures has been studied by Phariseau using Raman-Nath theory (see Ref. 3). He derived an important condition under which all but one diffraction order from the grating are suppressed. We may understand his important result by following a heuristic argument based on the first Born approximation.

Consider a single plane wave of light incident on a holographic grating from the direction given by the propagation vector $\vec{k}_i$ as shown in Fig. 4. The hologram contains an index of refraction which varies sinusoidally in amplitude, as shown, with planes of constant index normal to the surface of the hologram's emulsion. Then, it is well known (Viz. Carter, Ref. 5, Fig. 20) that the strongest order of diffracted light will be a single plane wave propagating in the direction given by the wave vector $\vec{k}_d$ in the figure where $\vec{K}_0$ is a vector directed normal to the planes of constant index in the hologram. This is essentially a phase matching condition for the light scattered from the various planes of constant index in the hologram. It is exactly analogous to the requirement for photon momentum conservation in quantum theory.

The scattering potential,

$$F(\vec{x}) = k^2 (n_0^2 - n^2(\vec{x})) \qquad (1)$$

represents the index of refraction variation from the minimum value n_0 inside of the hologram. $F(\vec{x})$ forms a Fourier transform pair with its angular spectrum in the form

$$F(\vec{x}) = \int\!\!\!\int_{-\infty}^{+\infty}\!\!\!\int \mathcal{A}(\vec{K}) \exp i(\pm \vec{K}\cdot\vec{x}) \, dK_y dK_z \qquad (2)$$

(see Carter, Ref. 5, Eq. (14)). Thus, for a usefully large class of functions $F(\vec{x})$ and $\mathcal{A}(\vec{K})$, we have the well

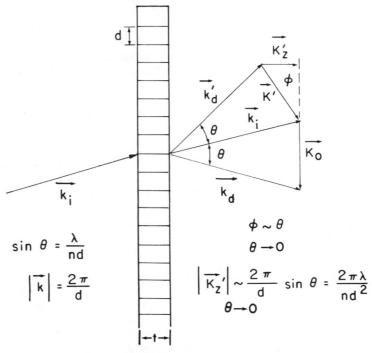

$$\sin \theta = \frac{\lambda}{nd}$$

$$|\vec{k}| = \frac{2\pi}{d}$$

$$\phi \sim \theta$$
$$\theta \to 0$$

$$|\vec{K_z'}| \sim \frac{2\pi}{d} \sin \theta = \frac{2\pi\lambda}{nd^2}$$
$$\theta \to 0$$

Fig. 4 — Diagram Illustrating the Notation.

known uncertainty relations

$$\Delta x \, \Delta K_x \geqslant 1$$
$$\Delta y \, \Delta K_y \geqslant 1 \qquad (3)$$
$$\Delta z \, \Delta K_z \geqslant 1$$

where Δx, Δy, Δz, and ΔK_x, ΔK_y, ΔK_z, represent the variances of $F(\vec{x})$ and $\mathscr{A}(\vec{K})$, respectively, along each of the Cartesian axes.

If we consider the effect of the thickness t of the hologram emulsion on $\vec{K}$, we see from Eq. (3) that $\Delta K_z \geqslant 1/t$. Furthermore, it is known from scattering theory in the first Born approximation that the amplitude of $\mathscr{A}(\vec{K}')$ is proportional to that of the plane wave of light diffracted into the direction $\vec{k}_d'$ which satisfies the phase matching conditions with $\vec{k}_i$ and $\vec{K}'$ (see Ref. 5, Eq. (30)). Finally, we can easily show from Eq. (2) that the finite thickness, t, gives rise to appreciable values of $\mathscr{A}(K)$ mainly over the range

$$|\vec{K}_z| < 1/t . \qquad (4)$$

Thus, Eq. (4) represents the condition for phase matching, i.e., for a diffracted plane wave with a propagation constant $\vec{k}_d'$ to be well phase matched, it must have associated with it a grating vector $\vec{K}' = \vec{k}_d' - \vec{k}_i$ which has a z-component $|\vec{K}_z'|$ less than $1/t$.

For small angles, Bragg's law can be expressed in the following form:

$$\sin \theta = N \, \frac{\lambda}{nd} \qquad (5)$$

which specifies all of the possible directions into which the incident plane wave can be diffracted, where N is an integer, θ is the full angle shown in the figure, and λ is the wavelength of the light. However, for these orders to actually occur they must also satisfy the phase matching condition. That is, the propagation vector $\vec{k}_d'$ must close with $\vec{k}_i$ and some vector $\vec{K}'$ for which the z-component satisfies Eq. (4). Thus, this order will be suppressed if

$$|K_z'| > 1/t . \qquad (6)$$

The phase matching condition for the diffraction order with the propagation constant $\vec{k}_d$ in Fig. 4 requires no z-component and will always occur. This is the first diffraction order that we will use for the output of the hologram as an optical element. The phase matching condition for one of the second diffraction orders with the propagation constant $\vec{k}_d'$ in Fig. 4 requires a z-component given in the limit as θ is made small by

$$|K_z'| = 2\pi\lambda/nd^2 . \qquad (7)$$

Thus by substitution from Eq. (7) into (6) we show that this diffraction order will not occur if the hologram is made thick enough so that

$$Q = 2\pi\lambda t/nd^2 > 1 \qquad (8)$$

where

t = emulsion thickness

d = grating spacing

n = index of refraction of gelatin.

The phase matching conditions for all of the higher diffraction orders require a still larger z-component for $\vec{K}$ and thus will also not occur if Eq. (8) is satisfied. This is Phariseau's condition which must be satisfied for an efficient hologram that will diffract almost all of the incident light into one desirable order. This theory, of course, neglects the effects of scattering due to an imperfect grating.

This derivation holds for small angles but we know from experimental work by Klein and others that for $Q \geqslant 10$ significant suppression of higher diffraction orders occurs (Ref. 6).

IV. EXPERIMENT

A. Proof-of-Concept

Some experiments have been conducted to establish proof-of-concept for using the two-step approach to making a hologram beam transformer.

For this proof-of-concept, we made the master hologram in Kodak 649F spectroscopic plates with 633 nm radiation from a He-Ne laser. To make this simulation more realistic, the grating spacing in the master hologram was limited to 4 microns, corresponding to the resolution limit of the IR sensitive IVN emulsion. The 4 micron grating period was obtained using the Mach-Zehnder interferometer shown in Fig. 5. One of the beams through the interferometer was used to simulate the astigmatic beam from the diode laser and the other simulated the well-collimated communications beam. A cylindrical lens was placed two focal lengths from the hologram plane in the simulated diode laser beam to produce astigmatism. The two beams were made to interfere at the hologram, and the plate was aligned so that the planes of constant index of refraction in the grating were normal to the surface of the emulsion. The exposure and processing were carried out using the Kodak recommendations for absorption holograms in 649F. The diffraction efficiency into the first order of these master holograms was found to be 9% to 10%.

The master hologram was copied into dichromated gelatin to create the working hologram. The plates were obtained from Dikrotek with an emulsion thickness of 13 ±1 microns. Efficient working holograms were obtained from the master holograms by greatly decreasing the grating period with the following copying method. The master hologram was reconstructed with a plane wave of 488 nm radiation from an Ar+ laser incident from a direction which maximized the brightness of one of the first order beams diffracted from the hologram. This order was made to interfere with a reference plane wave at the surface of the working hologram plate located two focal lengths of the cylindrical lens, now the hologram, from the plane of the master hologram as shown in Fig. 6. The angle of the reference beam relative to the

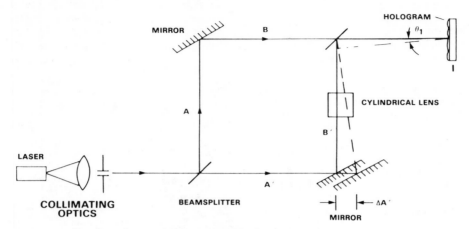

Fig. 5 — Diagram of the Apparatus for Constructing the "Master" Hologram.

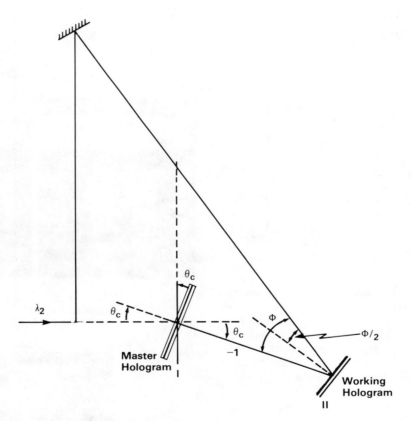

Fig. 6 — Diagram of Apparatus for Copying the "Master" Hologram into the Working Hologram.

beam reconstructed from the master hologram was varied to study the effect on the working hologram's efficiency. The dichromated gelatin holograms were developed with alcohol and water techniques specified by Dikrotek.

The developed working holograms made at 488 nm were reconstructed with 633 nm. A specific hologram was carefully aligned with the incident light beam to maximize the light intensity diffracted into the first order. The hologram efficiency into this first order and presence of other orders was noted as given in Table I. From the table, we notice that the working holograms were all quite efficient when reconstructed with 633 nm but that some of the holograms still produced observable higher orders. The number of observed orders decreased as Q was increased by increasing ϕ, as predicted. In the experiment described above, we were able to achieve high efficiencies using a 13 micron emulsion thickness with a grating spacing of about 1.2 microns, or a Q of 30.

Table I—Diffraction Efficiency into Observed Orders

EXPERIMENTAL RESULTS			
Q	0 (DEG)	ORDER	η (633 nm)
10	17.33°	+1	1.42%
		0	17.95
		−1	74.53
		−2	5.66
		−3	(nominal)
20	24.61	+1	.36
		0	10.0
		−1	87.86
		−2	1.43
30	30.26	0	4.85
		−1	94.0
35	32.75	0	5.42
		−1	93.60
40	35.08	0	7.72
		−1	91.90

$t \sim 13\mu$

We have not begun an investigation into the effect of aberrations induced by this technique, but by proper selection of recording and reconstructing geometries, it appears possible that for sufficiently thin emulsions, the wavefront reconstructed from the working hologram and working wavelength will be a replica with minimized aberrations of that which would have been constructed from the master hologram (Ref. 2).

B. IR Experiments

We examined several single-mode diode lasers for modal stability. Holograms are well known to be very sensitive to wavelength shifts so that it is important to use only well-stabilized lasers. An Ortel 20 mW laser diode was chosen as the most suitable for our initial experiments of those we tested.

To examine the coherence length, an interference pattern was observed through a CCD camera and video monitor using a Michelson interferometer as shown in Fig. 7. The interference patterns shown in Fig. 8 all reveal high contrast indicating high coherence. However, the observed patterns appear to contain speckle which we believe are due to reflections from the window inside the laser packaging. We will be experimenting with diodes with and without these windows in the future.

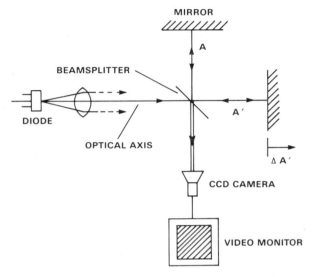

Fig. 7 — Diagram of the Apparatus for Measuring the Coherence Length of the Laser Diode Beam.

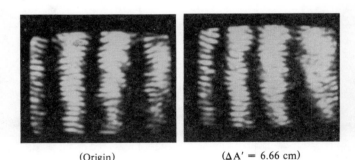

(Origin)   (ΔA' = 6.66 cm)

(a) Fringe Visibility and Contrast Comparison for Origin and Translated Path.

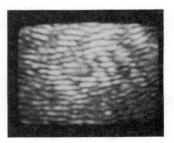

"Infrastructure"

(b) Speckle Pattern Evident Behind Coherence Fringes.

Fig. 8 — Interference Patterns from the Interferometer shown in Fig. 6.

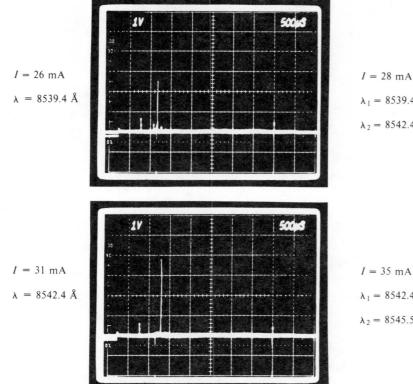

$I = 26$ mA

$\lambda = 8539.4$ Å

$I = 31$ mA

$\lambda = 8542.4$ Å

Fig. 9 — Diode Laser Mode Spectra Showing Regions of Modal Stability for the Ortel Laser Diode.

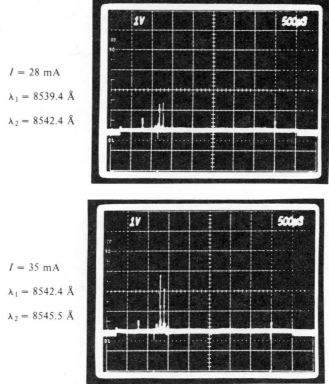

$I = 28$ mA

$\lambda_1 = 8539.4$ Å

$\lambda_2 = 8542.4$ Å

$I = 35$ mA

$\lambda_1 = 8542.4$ Å

$\lambda_2 = 8545.5$ Å

Fig. 10 — Diode Laser Mode Spectra Showing Regions of Modal Instability for the Ortel Laser Diode.

The spectra of the various diodes were observed using a Candela LS-1 laser spectrometer for various heat sink temperatures and current densities. We observed that under carefully controlled conditions, the Ortel single-mode laser diode could be made to operate with stability in a single mode as shown in the spectra in Figs. 9 and 10.

Some preliminary work was also done toward making master holograms in the IVN emulsion. We employed the Mach-Zehnder interferometer similar to that shown in Fig. 5. We have found the IVN material to be very sensitive at 854 nm so that very short times are required for proper hologram exposure. Energy densities on the order of 4 to 5 μJ/cm^2 are producing absorption holograms in this material, thereby precluding the need to pre-sensitize the plates. To date, we have been successful in making IR absorption holograms with grating periods of greater than 9.5 microns in the IVN emulsion.

V. CONCLUSIONS

We have demonstrated that holograms with at least 94% efficiency can be made in dichromated gelatin reconstructed at 633 nm. It is expected that equivalent results can be obtained for dichromated gelatin holograms that are made to be reconstructed at one of the diode laser wavelengths. To obtain the required efficiencies for a practical holographic beam corrector, two approaches appear to be viable. One may contact print a master holographic corrector into a thick dichromated gelatin emulsion. Alternatively, the master hologram may be copied by a two-step process which decreases the grating spacing thus permitting the use of thinner emulsions. Either approach offers the possibility of achieving highly efficient holograms with potentially minimized aberrations for operation in the near-Infrared.

Acknowledgement

The authors would like to thank Anne Clement and Ed Becker for their invaluable assistance in the laboratory during the course of the investigation of this problem.

REFERENCES

1. W.H. Carter and H.J. Caulfield, "Hologram Laser Beam Corrector and Combiner for a Satellite Data Link", Appl. Optics, 24, 2150 (1985).

2. C. Gilbreath-Frandsen and J.W. Wagner, "Holographic Optical Elements for Single-Mode Laser Diodes: A Practical Approach," Optics Letters (to be published).

3. P. Phariseau, "On the Diffraction of Light by Progressive Supersonic Waves," Proc. Ind. Acad. Sci. 44A, 165 (1956).

4. S.S. Duncan, J.A. McQuoid, D.J. McCarney, "Tunable holographic filters in dichromated gelatin operating in the near infrared region," Proc. SPIE, 523, 196 (1985).

5. W.H. Carter, "Three-dimensional Wave Theory of Optical Image Formation from Scattered Sound," J. Opt. Soc. Am. 60, 1366 (1970).

6. W.R. Klein, C.B. Tipnis, and E.A. Hiedemann, "Experimental Study of Fraunhofer Light Diffraction by Ultrasonic Beams of Moderately High Frequency at Oblique Incidence," Acoustica, 15, 229 (1965).

Session 3

Multiplexing in Holography

Chairmen
J. P. Huignard
Thomson CSF, France
B. Woodcock
Pilkington P.E. Ltd., United Kingdom

Two-dimensional optical beam
switching techniques using dynamic holography

G. PAULIAT and G. ROOSEN

INSTITUT D'OPTIQUE, Bât.503, Centre Universitaire d'Orsay
B.P. 43, 91406 ORSAY Cédex, FRANCE

J.P. HERRIAU, A. DELBOULBÉ and J.P.HUIGNARD

THOMSON CSF-LCR, Domaine de Corbeville, B.P. 10
91401 ORSAY, FRANCE

Abstract

A two dimensional optical switching device for fiber array has been investigated. The spatial commutation of an infrared beam from an optical fiber is produced in an entirely optical way : a photoinduced dynamic grating in a photorefractive crystal diffracts this beam assuring deflection in a given direction. Bragg condition is automatically matched. The large capacities thus obtained make this system attractive for its use in the optical networks.

Introduction

To assure commutation between fiber arrays, many different optical devices have been proposed. They are attractive because the connection is realized by a passive element.

Consequently they have no bandwidth limitation and are transparent to signal modulation. For small capacities opto_mechanical solutions are reliable {1}, but they seem not to be suitable for large ones {typically to assure commutation between 1000 x 1000 optical fibers}. For these cases opto optical systems appear to be more convenient {2,3,4}.

We describe here one of these techniques whose originality is to present a simple addressing method.

I. Basic principle of commutation with dynamic grating

In order to deflect a collimated infrared beam (at wavelength λ_o) from an optical fiber, a dynamic grating is placed on its path. A change in the fringe spacing Λ of this grating induces a variation of the emergence angle θ'_o of the diffracted beam producing commutation according to the relation : (see fig. 1).

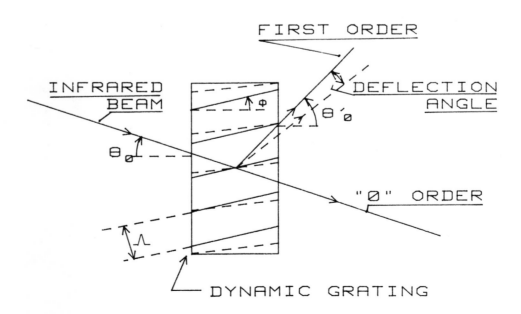

Fig.1. Basic principle of commutation with dynamic grating

$$\sin(\theta_o + \phi) - \sin(\theta'_o - \phi) = \pm \frac{\lambda_o}{N_o \Lambda} \quad (1)$$

where : θ_o is the incident angle of the beam

ϕ is the tilt of the fringe pattern

N_o is the refractive index

Actually,, the use of thick grating (wich allows better diffraction efficiency and only one diffracted order) requires to verify the Bragg condition {5} which is :

$$\theta_o - \phi \neq \theta'_o + \phi \quad (2)$$

It is easily seen form equations (1) and (2) that if we want to address several directions θ'_o we have to adapt simultaneously the two parameters $\Lambda(\theta'_o)$, $\phi(\theta'_o)$, according to :

$$\sin(\theta'_o - \phi(\theta'_o)) = \frac{\lambda_o}{2N_o \Lambda(\theta'_o)}$$

II. Addressing system with varying wavelength :

The dynamic grating is photoinduced in a material by two coherent plane waves from a dye laser (at wavelength λ). A fixed dispersive element is placed on the way of each of the writing beams (H_1, H_2 on figure 2).

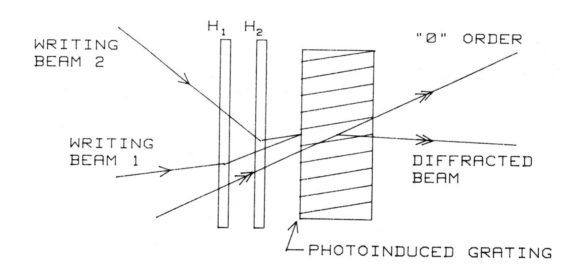

Fig. 2. Elementary compact switching cell using varying writing wavelength

So, by changing the wavelength λ, the incident angles of the recording beams upon the material are automatically modified.

Thus, a good choice of the dispersive elements allows to adapt simultaneously the set of two parameters Λ and ϕ. A variation of the addressing direction θ'_o is realized keeping maximum diffraction efficiency.

III. Choice of the components

i) Photosensitive material :

Photorefractive crystals are very attractive for this application for the following reasons :

+ They are available in great dimensions and high optical quality

+ The recording of the grating is made in the visible range with a total reversibility.

+ There is a memory effect : in the dark a photoinduced grating is recorded for several hours on days.

+ The diffraction of an infrared beam is nearly non destructive for the photoinduced grating. This, taking into account the memory effect, allows to maintain a connection even after the writing beams were turned off. These ones are then available to record a different grating to switch another infrared beam. By this way a single addressing system may be used to connect different lines.

Among all the photorefractive crystals, the Bismuth Silicon Oxide crystal, $Bi_{12} Si O_{20}$ (BSO) is chosen because of its sensitivity : an incident energy as low as 100 - 500 µJ cm^{-2} (at λ = 514,5 nm) is needed to write a grating {5}.

ii) Passive dispersive elements :

They are thick holographic gratings recorded in dichromated gelatin. They present high diffraction efficiency for the beam incident at Bragg angle {$\eta \neq 80\%$} but, for other beams they are transparent. Thus a very compact cell of commutation may be realized (figure 2).

IV. Experimental demonstration

Several elementary switching cells may be implemented and we have studied some of them {6}. The one here discussed has the following characteristics :

The infrared beam to deflect, at wavelength λ_o = 0,82 µm is incident at 30° on the crystal.

The crystal thickness is d = 2,74 mm.

The periods of the two holographic fixed gratings are P_1 = 1,5 µm and P_2 = 0,46µm.

The writing wavelength λ varies in the range {530 nm, 570 nm} and the average photoinduced fringe spacing is Λ = 2,6µm (at λ = 550 nm).

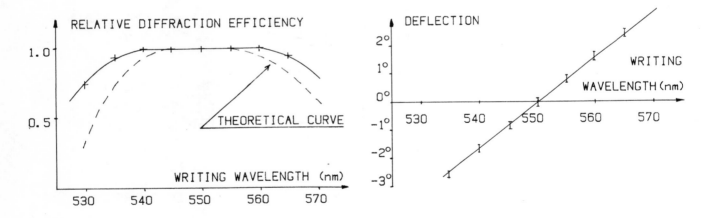

Fig. 3. Diffraction efficiency of an elementary switching all as a function of writing wavelength.

Fig. 4. Deflection of an Infrared beam as a function of writing wavelength.

The experimental relative efficiency is compared with the theoretical one on figure 3 and the corresponding deflection is represented on figure 4. A total deflection of 7° is obtained with a writing wavelength scan of 40nm. Considering the Rayleigh criterium, if the divergence of the incident beam is less than 1 mrd, then more than 130 different directions may be addressed.

To improve the absolute diffraction efficiency, an external electric field of 6 kV/cm is applied to the crystal. This efficiency is about 5.10^{-3}. However the use of average grating spacing of about 1 µm allows the working of the elementary cell without applied electric field. Such devices have been also studied and have given good results {6}.

V. Bi-dimensional deflection

If one the writing beam is moved out of the plan of figure 2, it results a rotation of the photoinduced grating. By this way, it is possible to deflect an infrared beam out of the plan of figure 2 and to produce a bidimensional deflection. This has been experimentally demonstrated by moving the writing beam by mechanical means. Deflections of about 4° have been obtained.

A proposal to realize this movement by means of electrooptical gates is made on figure 5. Each gate defines a direction of deflection perpendicular to those obtained by varying the writing wavelength as described in II.

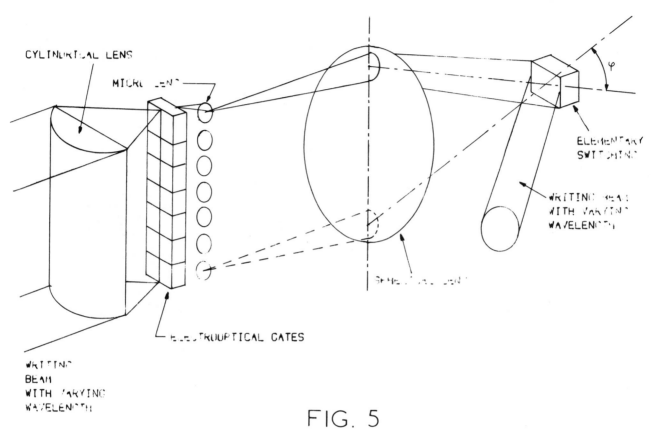

FIG. 5

V. Conclusions

The main features of this switching cell make it suitable for its use in optical networks. As seen above, a bidimensional device can easily address more than 32 x 32 = 1024 different directions. Thus a juxtaposition of several elementary cells can be implemented to swith 1024 x 1024 imput output.

The size of such a commutation plan may be as small as 10 x 10 cm^2 for single mode optical fibers. Thus, with the use of writing wavelength around λ = 500 nm and input power of a few watt, grating recording time constants of 200 ms may be obtained.

References

1. Jackel (J.L.), Hackwood (S), Beni (G), Appl. Phys. Lett. 40 (1), 1 January 1982.
2. P. Gravey and J. Lerouzic, Proceedings of IEE'84, May 1984.
3. J.P. Herriau, A. Delboulbé, B. Loiseaux, J.P. Huignard, J. Optics, 1984, Vol. 15, n° 5.
4. G.T. Sincerbox and G. Roosen, Applied Optics, Vol. 22, p. 690 (1983).
5. J.P. Huignard - F. Micheron, Appl. Phys. Lett. 29 - 591 - 1976.
6. G. Pauliat, J.P. Herriau, A. Delboulbé, G. Roosen, J.P. Huignard, Materials for Optical Processing feature, Josa B to be published in february 1986.

Holocoupler-Selfoc Fiber System: a coherent transfer matrix description

E. Guibelalde and M. L. Calvo[*]

Cátedra de Fisica Médica. Facultad de Medicina
*: Departamento de Optica. Facultad de Ciencias Fisicas
Universidad Complutense. 28040 Madrid. Spain

Abstract

The coupling in the Holocoupler-Selfoc fiber system is studied using a new matrix method, which may be applied to arbitrary x,y,z - varying structures. The properties of the spatial transfer function for invariant linear system are used.

Introduction

In previous works[1,2] the authors have developed a matrix method to obtain the transfer function of a general inhomogeneous optical medium presenting x,y,z varying structures.

The starting point of the method is the scalar wave equation. An exact integral equation is subsequently introduced in terms of a new propagator and iterative procedure are used. Further applications of Fourier Transform techniques lead to a matrix representation in which the coherent transfer function is obtained in terms of triangular matrices. The system is assumed to be linear. Those matrices characterize the reflection and transmission properties of the medium with arbitrary graded index profile. Some numerical stimates are presented in order to show the convergence and mathematical behaviour of the mentioned matrices. The dimensions of those matrices concide with the iteration number performed in the iterative procedure. The number of the representative matrix elements in the final transfer function depends on the physical parameters of the medium. The diagonal elements of the matrices represent the diffraction orders containing different amounts of energy.

The method has been developed for the particular case of an optical fiber with finite length and a parabolic index cross section and for different HOE´s. Among them, the case of a holographic lens is specially interesting. The coupling of the fiber[3] and lens can be directily studied assuming they are placed as in a linear cascade system[3].

The mentioned matrix method is related with other numerical methods as the Beam Propagation Method (BPM)[4,5].

General Formulation

If we consider a general profile of the form :

$$\varepsilon(x,y,z) = \varepsilon_0 (1 + \alpha\varepsilon_1(x,y,z)) \tag{1}$$

where ε_0 is the average dielectric constant and α is assumed to be a small modulation constant, we write the scalar wave equation in terms of the operator :

$$L = (\nabla^2 + k_0^2)^{1/2} \tag{2}$$

as :

$$(\partial^2 / \partial z^2 + L^2)\phi = - \alpha k_0^2 \varepsilon_1 \phi \tag{3}$$

where ∇^2 is the transverse laplacian operator and k_0 the free space propagation constant.

A complete solution of Equation 3 may be written in terms of the field at z = 0 as an integral equation :

$$\phi(x,y,z) = e^{-izL} \phi(x,y,0) - \alpha k_0^2 \int_0^z du \; \frac{\sin\{(z-u)\}}{L} \varepsilon_1(x,y,u) \; \phi(x,y,u) \tag{4}$$

After performing a Fourier Transform over Equation 4 and taking some far-field approximation over the iterative solution we can write the scalar field as :

$$FT\{\phi(x,y,z)\} = H(f_x,f_y,z) \cdot FT\{\phi(x,y,0)\} \tag{5}$$

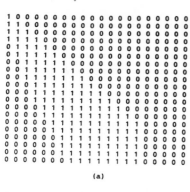

(a)

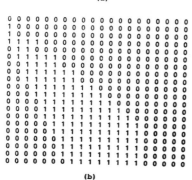

(b)

Figure 1. Digital simulation of
a fiber optic characte-
ristic matrix.

where H is a generalized transfer function which depends now on an algebraic operator:

$$A = (k_0^2 - 4\pi^2 f^2)^{1/2} \qquad (6)$$

and fulfills the general properties of the transfer
function:

1.- $H(0,0,0) = 1$
2.- $H(-f_x,-f_y,-z) = H^*(f_x,f_y,z)$
3.- $|H(f_x,f_y,z)| \leq |H(0,0,0)|$

The developed transfer function for a slightly variant medium with the coordinate z is of the form :

$$H(f_x,f_y,d) = \bar{B}\{e^{-iAd} M_{pxp}^T + e^{iAd} M_{pxp}^R\}\bar{D} \qquad (7)$$

where $\bar{B}$ and $\bar{D}$ are p-dimensional vectors containing,
respectively, information about the optical properties of the medium and about the thickness. M^T and
M^R are triangular matrices which characterize the
transmission and reflection properties of the medium.
P is the number of iterations performed in the integral equation.

In Figure 1 a digital simulation is presented to
show a distribution of the non-negligeable elements
of the characteristic matrices of an optical fiber
(length d = 1m. and α = 1E-2). The 1-elements are
larger than 1E-7.

Transfer Function of a Selfoc Fiber

The coherent transfer function of a Selfoc fiber can be obtained assuming a dielectric
constant of the form :

$$\varepsilon(\rho) = \begin{cases} \varepsilon_0\{1 + (2\Delta/1-2\Delta).(1-(\rho/R)^2)\} & 0 \leq \rho \leq R \\ \varepsilon_0 & \rho \geq R \end{cases} \qquad (8)$$

where ρ is the radius, $\rho = (x^2+y^2)^{1/2}$, ε_0 represents a dielectric constant of an infinite
extended cladding and R the core radius. The wavelength of the incoming light is suppose to
be 1µm and $\alpha = 2\Delta/1-2\Delta$ is a small parameter.

The coherent transfer function of
this profile can be obtained using
the characteristic matrix method.

The results, using a 20x20 transmission characteristic matrix is
shown in Figure 2. There, the real
and imaginary parts of H appear.
f is the spatial frequency.

Calculations were performed for
a 25µm core radius, which corres-
pons to a tipical multimode fiber.
In this figure a divergent behaviour
is observed at f = 1000 lp/mm. That
corresponds to plane waves propagating transversally to the axis. Larger frequencies will give waves similar to the evanescent ones.

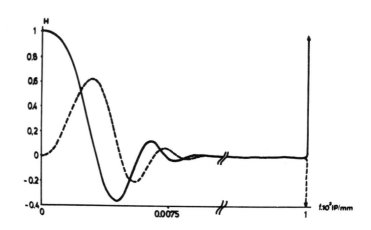

Figure 2. Cont. line : Real part of H^T.
Dotted line: Imaginary part of H^T

Figures 3 and 4 represent, respectively, the modulus and phase of the transfer function. If the effect of the angular spectrum in free space (Figure 5) is included, the real part of the phase term takes the form presented in Figure 6. Finally, in Figure 7, a tridimensional picture of H^T is shown.

The execution time for a 20x20 computation grid was 7.30 minutes and the required time for performing the 20x20 characteristic matrix was 35 seconds.

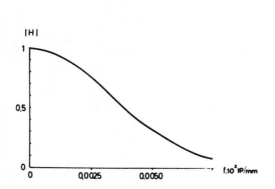

Figure 3. Modulus of H^1. The first cut-off frequency is obtained at 10lp/mm.

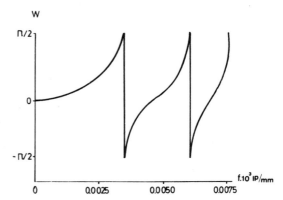

Figure 4. Phase distorsion term obtained for a parabolic profile.

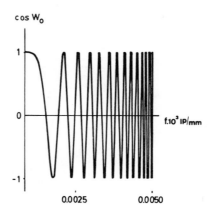

Figure 5. Propagation of the free space angular spectrum

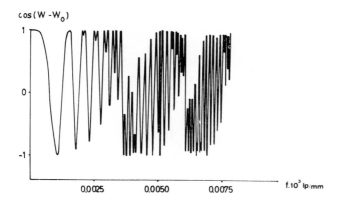

Figure 6. Real part of the phase distorsion term modulated by the angular spectrum of free space.

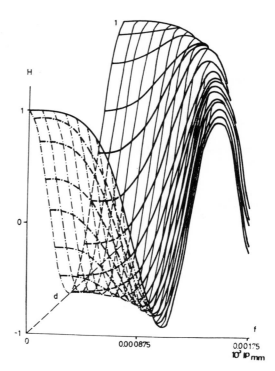

Figure 7. 3-D representation of H^T in terms of the length of the optical fiber and spatial frequency. One pulse is represented.

Transfer Function of a Holographic Lens

The dielectric constant variation of a holographic lens formed by interfering plane and spherical scalar waves can be written as :

$$\varepsilon(x,y,z) = \varepsilon_0 \left(1 + \frac{\alpha}{r} \cos\{\beta(r-z)\} \right) \tag{9}$$

with :

$$r = \left(x^2 + y^2 + (z_0+z)^2 \right)^{1/2} \tag{10}$$

z_0 is the focal length of the lens and β the forming wavelength of the hologram.

If a large focal length is considered, $z_0 \gg x,y,z$, a new profile can be used to represent the holographic lens:

$$\varepsilon(x,y,z) = \varepsilon_0 \left(1 + \frac{\alpha}{z_0} \cos\{\beta/z_0((x^2 + y^2)^{1/2} + z^2)\} \right) \tag{11}$$

an exact solution for the transmission field can be developed using a matrix method. The condition that neglects the reflected field is :

$$\frac{d}{z_0} \ll 4 \frac{k_0}{\beta}(1 - (2\pi f/k_0)^2)^{1/2} \tag{12}$$

where d is the thickness of the lens ans f the spatial frequency. In Figure 8 the condition (Equation 12) is shown for different rates k_0/β. It can be noticed that, e.g. a lens of $z_0 = 1$ mm. and $d = 10\mu m$ fulfills the condition.

The final transfer function of the holographic lens using the matrix method takes the form of an exponential :

$$H^T_{lens}(f,d) = e^{-W} \exp\{i(Ad-W')\} \tag{13}$$

with W and W' functions of Fresnel integrals. This transfer function is a generalized amplitude and phase filter.

The modulation of amplitude by the cos of the phase is presented if Figure 9. It is noticeable that the parabolic effect appears for f < 12.5 lp/mm.

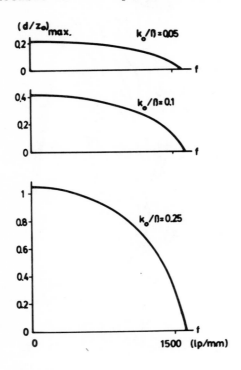

Figure 8. Frequency zones and maximum of d/z_0 values for a lens as a transmission HOE in terms of k_0/β.

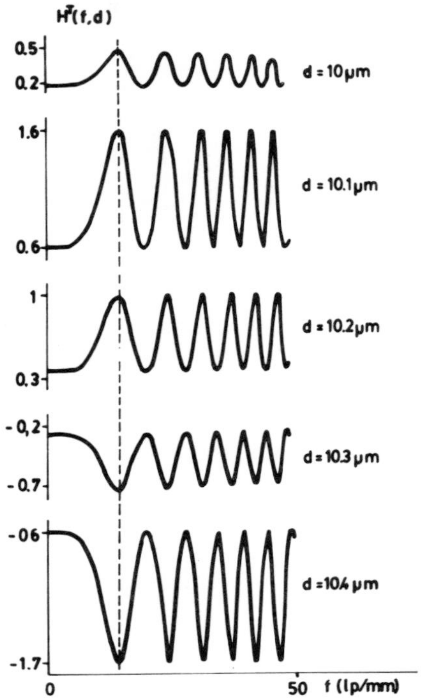

Figure 9. Transfer function of a holographic lens for different thickness. The dotted line shows the parabolic behaviour zone.

Coupling Transfer Function of the cascade system

One of the most important advantage of our mathematical analysis is the possibility of being used in different optical devices. Thus, it finds a clear application in the study of propagation through linear cascade system using the properties of transfer functions.

The generalized expression for the solution of the cascade system will be :

$$FT\{\Phi(x,y,z)\} = H_1 \, H_2 \, H_3 \, \cdots \cdots \, FT\{\Phi(x,y,0)\} \qquad (14)$$

where H_i is the transfer function of GRIN i.

In Figure 10, the coupling between the modulii of the fober transfer function and lens transfer function is shown. As it can be noticed, the transfer function of the lens is cut in the parabolic zone of Figure 9. In this frequency zone there are no distorsion introduced in the fiber and a loss in the confined energy of approximately 25% is observed.

Finally, in Figure 11 the cosenus of the phase term for the coupling system is shown and in Figure 12 the final coupling transfer function:

$$H_{coupling} = |H_{fiber}| \cdot |H_{lens}| \cdot \cos(W' - A(d_f + d_1)) \qquad (15)$$

Conclusions

The coupling of GRIN media is studied using a new matrix method which may be applied to x,y,z varying structures. Using the properties of spatial transfer functions for invariant linear systems, the loss energy and profile distorsion are evaluated for the coupling system: Holographic lens-Selfoc fiber.

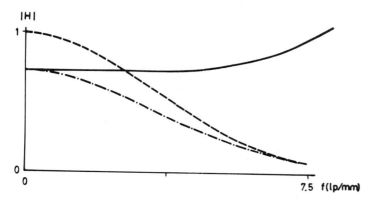

Figure 10. Modulus coupling between the
transfer functions.
Dotted line : |H FIBER|
Cont. line : |H LENS|
.-.-.- line : |H COUPLING|

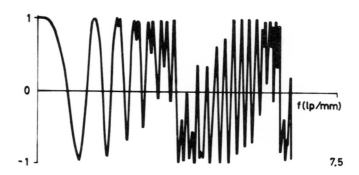

Figure 11. Phase term of the coupling.

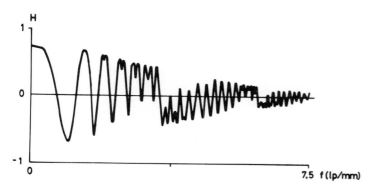

Figure 12. Transfer function of the coupling system: Holographic lens
- Selfoc fiber.

References

1. Guibelalde,E. and Calvo,M.L., "Reflection and Transmission Characteristic Matrices for the spatial impulse response of a graded index optical medium", Proc.ICO-13 Conf.Digest Ed.H.Ozhu 1984, pp. 708-709.

2. Guibelalde,E. and Calvo,M.L., "Coherent and incoherent illumination in optical fibers: A transfer matrix description for the transmission and reflection of light", Acta Polyt.Sc. Appl.Phys.Series., Vol.149, pp.245-248. 1985.

3. Gaskill, J.D., Linear System, Fourier Transform and Optics, John Wiley & Sons 1978.

4. Feit, M.D. and Fleck, J.A., "Light propagation in graded index optical fibers", Appl.Optics, Vol.17, pp.3990-3998. 1978.

5. Yevick, D. and Thylen, J., "Analysis of gratings by the Beam Propagation Method", J.Opt.Soc.Am., Vol. 72, pp.1084-1089. 1982.

Holographic optical element wavelength multi-demultiplexer
in the near infrared

De Schryver F.M.

Université Libre de Bruxelles, Service des Milieux Continus,
CP 194/5, Av. F. Roosevelt, 50; 1050 Bruxelles, Belgium.

Abstract.

Two methods performing wavelength division multiplexing or wavelength division demultiplexing in the near infrared region and using volume transmission holographic optical element are presented. In the first one, the holographic optical element converts collimated light beams (output beam of optical fiber coupled with a GRIN lens) and the second method handles direct output beam of the fiber. Advantages and drawbacks of the methods are investigated.

Introduction.

Considerable interest has recently been shown in the use of wavelength division multiplexing and wavelength division demultiplexing devices (WDM-WDD)[1]. These devices are very attractive from the view point of their flexibility and are also interesting to increase the capacity of optical fiber transmission systems by sending simultaneously signals having different wavelengths and precise bandwidth, using the wide low loss wavelength range of an optical fiber. This eliminates the need of multiple fibers or allows increased capacity on existing networks and cost reduction.

Optical WDM-WDD are generally classified into two types: wavelength selective and wavelength non-selective [1] (like directionnal or polarization couplers). The wavelength selective type is splitted in passive and active types (multiwavelength light sources and detectors). The passive type is further made up of dielectric thin film filter (DTF), angular dispersive elements and hybrid system (DTF + angular dispersive). Angulary dispersive elements have the advantage of compactness and the possibility to handle a large number of different channels. The key element in such device is an angulary dispersive element like a prism or a grating (in Czerny - Turner or Littrow configuration) or a concave surface diffraction grating.

In addition to those devices, a transmission volume holographic optical element (HOE) recorded in dichromated gelatin (DCG) can be used to perform the requirements and we present in this paper the successive stages for its conception and its fabrication.

HOE as WDM-WDD.

Transmission volume HOE have several advantages to use as WDM-WDD[2]:
- in the case of a phase lossless grating (conductivity σ=o), a high diffraction efficiency can be reached (theoretically 100%) for a given wavelength.
- the dispersion in intrinsically high and the bandwidth can be adjusted to obtain a narrow or a broad bandpass. If a broad bandpass is choosen, a large number of wavelengths can be handled by such device. In the present case, the device will be designed to handle 4 different wavelengths (1240, 1270, 1300 and 1330 nm) and will be tested at 1300 nm.

The photosensitive material used for the construction of the HOE is the DCG. Up to now, DCG is one of the best materials for holographic recording because high diffraction efficiencies can be obtained (experimental results between 70 and 95% can be typically reached), it is possible to have up to 8% for the modulation of the index of refraction, variable thicknesses of the gelatin, low scattering, high resolution and high damage threshold. One major problem is that DCG is sensitive only in the blue-green region of the spectrum. As the wavelengths of interest are located in the infrared, the geometry of the set-up during the reconstruction step will differ from that of the recording.

Two different recording configurations can be considered[8]:
- a HOE constructed by interference between plane waves
- a HOE constructed by interference between a converging and a diverging spherical beam.

For the reconstruction, in the case of the conversion between plane waves, a collimating lens must be positionned at the output of the emitting and receiving fiber (fig2b). This additionnal element is a limitation of the device because supplementary insertion losses must be taken in account. In the case of a conversion between spherical waves, direct light beam emitted by the input fiber can be used to illuminate the HOE and the diffracted beam can be directly injected in the receiving fiber. The advantage of this last configuration is that no other element than the HOE is needed to complete the injection, and consequently, the coupling losses are minimized provided the numerical aperture of the HOE corresponds to that of the fiber and the readout geometry minimizes the aberrations induced by the change of geometry.

HOE operating with collimated light.

1.Theory.

In a volume HOE, several parameters affect the diffraction efficiency, the bandwidth, and the dispersion. Those parameters must be appropriated to give high diffraction efficiency in the range of the wavelengths selected for the utilization.
The figure 1 represents a general schematic view of the recording set-up.

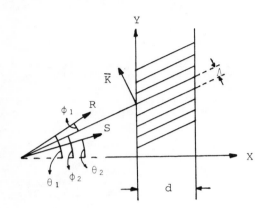

Figure 1.

R: Reference wave; S: Signal wave; $\overline{K}$: grating vector
d: thickness of emulsion; Λ: fringes spacing.

The diffraction efficiency can be derived from the coupled wave theory and is given by[3]:

$$\eta = \frac{\sin^2 \sqrt{\nu^2 + \xi^2}}{1 + (\xi^2/\nu^2)}$$

where

$$\nu = \pi\, n_1\, d\, /\lambda\, \sqrt{C_r C_s}$$

n_1 is the amplitude of modulation for the index of refraction, $C_r \approx \cos\theta_1$, $C_s \approx \cos\theta_2$ are obliquity factors.

and

$$\xi = \xi_{\Delta\lambda} + \xi_{\Delta\theta}$$

is an "off-Bragg parameter", with

$$\xi_{\Delta\theta} = \Delta\theta\, 2\pi\, n_1\, d\, \sin\theta/\,\lambda \qquad \text{and} \quad \xi_{\Delta\lambda} = \Delta\lambda\, 2\pi\, n_1\, d\, \sin^2\theta\, /\, \lambda^2\, \cos\theta$$

In the Bragg condition, $\xi = 0$ and the optimum value to obtain a maximum diffraction efficiency is $\nu = \pi/2$.
As, for a given angle, only one wavelength will satisfy the Bragg law, the bandwidth and the dispersion of the HOE must also be taken in account to keep an optimum diffraction efficiency for the other wavelengths.
The bandwidth for a transmission hologram is[7]:

$$\frac{\Delta\lambda}{\lambda} = \frac{\sqrt{3}\Lambda}{2d\, \text{tg}\theta} \qquad (\theta_1 = -\theta_2 = \theta \text{ for an unslanted grating } \phi_2 = 0)$$

To determinate the angular dispersion, we derive the Bragg condition to obtain:

$$\Delta\theta = \Delta\lambda\, /\, n\, \Lambda\, \cos\theta$$

As it can be observed, it is advantageous to choose to have a wide bandwidth (to have an optimum diffraction efficiency) but it is also necessary to have a maximum angular dispersion (for the positionning of the receiving fibers). It is therefore indispensable to find a compromise between both conditions.
As the HOE is symmetrical, it can operate both ways: R→S or S→R, i.e. demultiplexing or multiplexing wavelengths; further on, we will consider only the demultiplexing function.

2.Experiments.

The recording set-up is that of figure 2a.

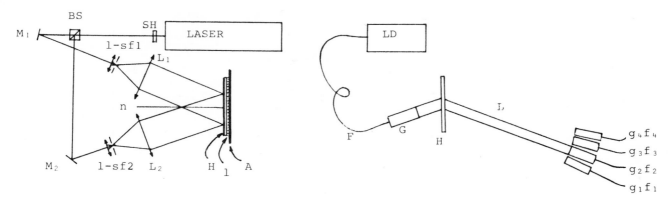

Figure 2a.

Figure 2b.

BS: beam-splitter; M_1, M_2: mirrors
l-sf1,2: lens-spatial filter assembly;
L_1,L_2: collimating lenses; H: hologram
l: index matching fluid; A: absorber.

LD: laser diode (1.3 μm); F: input
fiber; G, g_1,g_2,g_3,g_4: GRIN lenses;
H: hologram; f_1,f_2,f_3,f_4: output fibers.

The light of an argon laser (λ=488 nm) is separated in two by means of a variable beam splitter; the two beams are expended and filtered by the l-sf assemblies, collimated by the lenses L_1 and L_2 and finally interfere on the photosensitive plate H with gelatin side facing. Each beam makes an angle α relative to the normal n of the plate. An absorber is placed behind the plate H and the interstice is filled with an index matching liquid to avoid parasitical reflections. After the exposition, controlled with the electronic shutter SH, the photoplate is processed following the standard procedure [4]. The thickness of the emulsion is 15 μm.
The calculated incidence angle in the gelatin is θ=5°79 (in the air, α=8°82). This conducts to a fringe spacing of 1.59 μm. The calculated full bandwidth is 429 nm and the angular deviation for a wavelength change of 30 nm is 13 10^{-3} rad. If we desire to have a spacing between the center of two adjacent output beams of 1 mm (diameter of a GRIN lens), a distance L=9 cm is necessary behind the HOE for the positionning of the receiving fibers.

For the reconstruction (figure 2b), the HOE is tested using a laser diode source (λ = 1300 nm) with a 50 / 125 μm fiber pigtail. A GRIN lens (Selfoc type) is fixed at the extremity of the input fiber F to obtain a collimated beam illuminating the HOE at Bragg angle. The diffraction efficiency is measured by a photodiode (Anritsu MA 96 A) coupled with a power meter (Anritsu ML 93 A) directly positionned in the diffracted beam. The expression of the diffraction efficiency is choosen as:

$$\eta = I_1 /(I_1 + I_0)$$

where I_1 is the intensity of the diffracted beam and I_0 is the intensity of the transmitted beam. So, the losses due to the reflected beam are automatically taken in account (and, in fact, could be eliminated if the whole set-up was imerged in a tank filled with index matching liquid). Diffraction efficiency of around 80% is measured.
As the necessary distance behind the hologram is relatively large and the beam emerging of the GRIN lens is not perfectly collimated but is slightly diverging, the insertion loss due to the receiving GRIN lens is important; a way to solve that problem is to use a HOE recorded between a slightly diverging and a slightly converging beams (for reference and signal beams respectively) to compensate the divergence of the reconstructing beam and the insertion loss of the system can fall around 2 dB.

HOE operating with spherical beams.

1.Theory.

The hologram is now fabricated by recording the interferences between a spherical diverging beam and a spherical converging beam. The general case will de envisaged, when, during the reconstruction step, the hologram is illuminated by a sherical diverging beam which is in a location and has a wavelength different from those of recording. To calculate the diffraction efficiency, the principle is to apply localy the coupled wave theory where the grating is supposed to be unidimensionnal and then, integrate over the entire hologram. The diffraction efficiency can be written as [5]:

$$\eta = \frac{\int I_R(P)\ \eta(P)\ d\sigma}{\int I_R(P)\ d\sigma}$$

where $I_R(P)$ is the field intensity of a reconstructing spherical wave illuminating the HOE at the point P, and σ is the integration variable.

$\eta(P)$ is the local conversion efficiency in the vicinity of the point P which depends on the amplitude of modulation of the index of refraction, d/λ, the ratio between the wavelength during the recording and that of the reconstruction, and also on geometrical parameters as the off axis angle, the numerical aperture of the HOE, the distance of the reference point source during the recording and that of the reconstruction to the center of the HOE, and the distance of the reconstructed signal point to the center of the HOE.

Another important point is the problem of the minimization of the aberrations [6]. These aberations are caused by the mismatching of three wavefronts: the reference and signal beams used for the recording and the reconstruction wavefront. Indeed, generally, the reconstruction source has a location and a wavelength different of that of the recording reference source. The aberrations are separated in chromatic type (due to the change of wavelength) and geometric type (due to the change of position); further, the geometric type can be separated in spherical, comatic and astigmatic type. Several computer programs exist to minimize those aberrations and are helpfull for the design of the HOE.

Finally, the bandwidth and the angular dispersion have still to be analyzed for the same reasons than for the first HOE type.

2. Experiments.

The experimental set-up is that of figure 3a for the recording step.

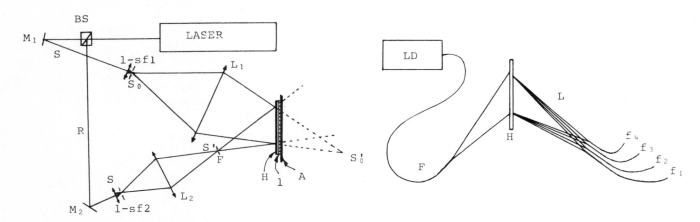

Figure 3a.

Figure 3b.

BS: beam-splitter; M_1, M_2: mirors;
1-sf1,2: lens-spatial filter assembly;
L_1, L_2: converging lenses; H: hologram;
1: index matching liquid; A: absorber.
R: reference; S: signal.

LD: laser diode (1.3 m); F: input fiber; H: hologram; f_1, f_2, f_3, f_4: output fibers.

The beam of the argon laser is separated in two by means of the beam splitter. The signal beam point source S_0 is imaged through the lens L_1 to give rise to the image point S_0'. The reference beam point source is imaged through the lens L_2 and gives rise to the source S_r' spatially filtered (F). This configuration was necessary to avoid encumbrance problems. The two beams interfere finally on the photoplate, the optical axis of each beam making an angle α relative to the normal n of the plate. The thickness of the emulsion was 15 μm.

The calculated incidence angle in the gelatin is 12°5 (in the air, $\alpha=19°2$). This gives rise to a fringe spacing of 0.74 μm. The calculated full bandwidth is 251 nm and the angular deviation for a wavelength change of 30 nm is 27 mrad. As the dispersion is more important in this case than before and as no GRIN lenses are necessary, the length behind the HOE is reduced to 2 cm, for a separation of 0.5 mm for two adjacent reconstructed image points.

For the reconstruction (figure 3b), the HOE is tested using the laser diode emitting at 1.3 µm. The output ligth of the 50/125 µm fiber pigtail illuminates the HOE under the best possible incidence angle. The diffraction efficiency is measured by a photodiode positionned directly in the diffracted beam. The expression of the diffraction efficiency is the same as before. Values around 75% are obtained. The insertion loss of the complete system is currently studied.

Conclusion.

The feasibility of constructing a transmission volume holographic optical element for use in the near infrared has been demonstrated. Diffraction efficiencies of 80% were reported in the case of conversion between plane waves. An application to wavelength division demultiplexing has also been proposed.

Acknowledgments.

The author wishes to thank A.C.E.C. (E.A.T. division) and I.R.S.I.A. for their financial support.

References.

1.Hikedi Ishio, Junichiro Minowa, Kiyoshi Nosu :Review and status of wavelength division multiplexing technology and its applications, Journal of Lightwave Technology, vol. LT-2, n°.4, p.448, 1984.

2.J.L. Horner, J.E. Ludman : Single holographic element wavelength demultiplexer Applied Optics, vol.20, n°.10, p.1845, 1981.

3.H. Kogelnik : Coupled wave theory for thick hologram gratings, Bell System Tech. Journal, 48, p.2909, 1969.

4.B.J. Chang, D. Leonard : Dichromated gelatin for the fabrication of holographic optical elements, Applied Optics, vol.18, n°.14, p.2407, 1979.

5.H. Nishihara : Efficiency of a holographic wavefront converter, Applied Optics vol.21, n°.11, p.1995, 1982.

6.J.N. Latta : Computer based analysis of hologram imagery and aberrations, Applied Optics, vol.10, n°.3, p.599, 1971 and p.609, 1971.

7.L. Solymar, D.J. Cooke : Volume holography and volume gratings, Academic Press, 1981.

8.M.A. Corbusier : Engineer thesis, sevice des milieux continus, University of Brussel, 1985.

A new holographic interferometer with monomode fibers for integrated optics applications

Torsten von Lingelsheim and Thomas Ahrens

Institut für Hochfrequenztechnik der TU Braunschweig
P.O.Box 3329, D-3300 Braunschweig, Germany (FRG)

Abstract

A new holographic interferometer concept for novel applications in integrated optic grating device manufacturing has been developed. The spatial filters have been substituted by two special monomode fibers with a core diameter below 5 μm. Only the finite size of the fiber mounts limits now the beam interference angle, thus leading to great flexibility in design of the desired curved or chirped grating groove formation.

Introduction

Many integrated optic devices such as duplexers, multiplexers, demultiplexers or filters consist in their main part of a small grating area with a corrugated surface.[1] Usually, this surface is formed by a photolithographic process using photosensitive resist and holographic exposure equipment. For some new WDM components it is important to manufacture curved or chirped gratings.[2,3] Unfortunately, the usual holographic equipment is insufficient in this case, because of the large physical dimensions of the optical and mechanical components in comparison to the small exposure area. It becomes impossible to make the necessary geometrical arrangements of the components, in particular of the closely spaced spatial filter mounts to obain low angle interference.

Therefore, a new holographic interferometer concept for applications in I.O. device manufacturing processes has been developed. The spatial filters have been substituted by two special monomode fibers with a core diameter below 5 μm. Their core areas act as point sources for the formation of the interference pattern. Due to the small fiber mounts a greater flexibility of the geometrical arrangement and, thereby, of the desired groove formation can be achieved.

Some of the problems arising in connection with interfering gaussian beams as emitted by the fibers have been solved by calculation. First samples of chirped grating areas have been manufactured and measured. They confirm the possibilities of this fiber-optic interferometer for I.O. applications.

Theoretical investigations

Fig. 1 shows the general configuration of the fiber-optic interferometer. A He-Cd laser beam is divided into two rays by a variable beam splitter ST. Each of the beams is focussed with a microscope objective (20 x, 0.35) to the core region of a monomode fiber MF, which is attached to the adjustable fiber mount FH. The fibers are then guided through mode strippers MS filled with liquid paraffin. Additional fiber clamps K protect the fibers against physical damage on the vibration isolated optical bench. The adjustable fiber clamp not only protects the fiber, but also by inducing controlled stress, can help to reduce problems due to polarization change in the conical fiber output beams. The fiberends are attached to special fiber mounts FH of the exposure equipment. The arrangement of this exposure equipment allows great variations for the adjustment of interference angle and exposure distance. A few details of the actual interferometer device will be given in a later section of this contribution.

The theoretical investigations are based on the geometrical quantities as defined in Fig. 2. The monomode fibers 1 + 2, whose cores act as point sources in this interferometric configuration, are located in a x-y-plane symmetrically to the y-axis at $-x_0$ and $+x_0$, respectively. The extended fiber axes intersect the y-axis at y_0. The plane of exposure is perpendicular to the x-y-plane, intersects the y-axis at y_s and makes an angle γ with the x-axis. The calculation of the constructive and destructive phase behavior of this general interference problem was based on.[4] For the two beams the respective phase shifts by the path lengths to a point A on the ξ-axis are calculated. The loci of constructive interference at $z = 0$ can then be calculated from:

$$\xi_m = \frac{a^2 y_s \tan\gamma}{c^2 - a^2 (1+\tan^2\gamma)} + \sqrt{\left[\frac{a^2 y_s \tan\gamma}{c^2 - a^2 (1+\tan^2\gamma)}\right]^2 + \frac{a^2 (c^2 - a^2 + y_s^2)}{c^2 - a^2 (1+\tan^2\gamma)}} \qquad (1)$$

$$\text{with} \quad a = m\lambda/2$$
$$c = y_s \tan\alpha_o$$
$$m = 0, \pm 1, \pm 2, \ldots$$

The distance between adjacent maxima of intensity in the exposure plane, also known as the grating constant, follows as:

$$d_m = \xi_{(m+1)} - \xi_m \qquad (2)$$

For the extensions of the fiber axes intersecting on the exposure plane at $y_s = y_o$ the results of the calculations are depicted in Figs. 3a-c. Fig. 3a shows the grating constant d_m as function of the number of maxima m with the interference angle α_o as parameter. The relatively small variations of only 5 % of α_o change the grating constant between 5.7 μm and 6.3 μm. Fig. 3b shows the dependence of d_m on the distance parameter y_o. One can see that a variation of y_o changes the chirp rate especially in the outer interference region. Furthermore, the misalignment angle γ of the exposure plane leads to asymmetrical curves for the grating constant (Fig. 3c). The interference behavior of the fiber-optic interferometer can be summarized as follows:

1) The grating constant is mainly determined by the interference angle α_o. Its values in the center for $m = o$ are shown in Fig. 4.

2) The chirp behavior of the grating constant depends mainly on y_o.

3) A rotation of the exposure plane (e.g. by a misalignment of the equipment) leads to an asymmetric shift of the curves for the grating constant.

For the photoresist development process only the power distribution in the exposure plane is important. The Fig. 5 shows the additional removal Δd of the resist AZ 1350 versus the applied energy E.[5] This development characteristic of the resist allows a qualitative prediction of the process. Two characteristic points can be defined. Below 30 mJ/cm2 of applied exposure energy no significant removal occurs during the development process. Above 130 mJ/cm2 the resist removal is independent of the applied energy, the development process is saturated. Therefore, in all cases an intensity ratio greater than 4.33 must be achieved by the intensities of constructive and destructive interference to ensure suitable development conditions for the grating structure. For numerical calculations of the resulting intensity from both interfering laser beams we used the holographic equation[6] (see Fig. 2 for reference):

$$I_{res} = I_1 + I_2 + 2\sqrt{I_1 I_2} \cos\left\{2\pi \frac{(r_2 - r_1)}{\lambda}\right\} \qquad (3)$$

With I_1 and I_2 as the intensities and r_1 and r_2 as distances between the fiber endface and a point A on the plane of exposure, respectively. Furthermore, we assumed Gaussian beams according to

$$\frac{I_{1,2}(\beta)}{I_o} \sim \exp\left\{-\frac{\beta_{1,2}^2}{\beta_{max}}\right\} \qquad (4)$$

with β_{max} as the cone angle of the radiated beam. To ensure homogeneous development characteristics across the whole grating area the difference of available energy in the interference maxima should not exceed 15 %. For these conditions Fig. 6 shows the diameter D of the predicted exposure area as function of the normalized distance y_o/y_s. Within the circle of this diameter no major problems occur. With special care in the exposure and development procedure an intensity variation up to 32 % can be tolerated and leads to still adequate results. For our requirements we had no need to extend the exposure area any further.

Device performance

The two main important parts of the actual device, the exposure equipment and the monomode fiber, will now be discussed in detail. Fig. 7 depicts the exposure equipment. To the left and to the right the mode stripping paraffin pots are located. The v-like part in the center is the angle position mechanism with its special sliding fiber mount containing height and rotation adjustment facilities. The samples are attached to a micropositioner-controlled exposure plane by a vacuum chuck. The remaining parts of the interferometer are standard holographic equipment.

The fabrication of a suitable monomode fiber was a problem from the start of the project. Optical requirements for this fiber are as follows:

1) The fiber must be single mode at 441.6 nm (He-Cd laser wavelength).

2) The core diameter should be as small as possible to satisfy the "point source" condition.

3) The numerical aperture should be as large as possible in order to increase the area of useful interference.

The profile of the most suitable fiber for our application, as measured by the refractive nearfield method, is drawn in Fig. 8. F-doping during the MCVD-preform-manufacturing process leads to a depressed refractive index ring around the core region. This increases the relative refractive index difference Δ by 0.074 % to 0.214 %. With a core diameter of 4.2 μm the LP_{11} cut-off wavelength of this fiber is 350 nm. To characterize the samples manufactured with this interferometer equipment, Fig. 9 shows the nearly flawless interference pattern of a photoresist grating after exposure, development and deposition of a thin gold layer.

In order to measure the expected very small grating constant variations of the order of 1 nm, we developed a computerized measurement test set, which is schematically shown in Fig. 10. The grating under test is mounted exactly normal to an incident He-Ne laser beam. This position is controlled by the retroreflection of the gratings 0th order. Then, the angle α between this 0th order and the 1st order is measured very precisely with the distance s as determined by a quadrant detector (accuracy 12 μm) which itself is moved by a stepper motor with a resolution of 1000 steps for each full rotation. The computer collects all data and calculates the grating constant for the illuminated point on the grating surface. To reduce additional errors arising from random last bits of the stepper motor or from vibration problems as caused by the rotating mechanics, each measurement has been repeated several times and evaluated statistically. Fig. 11 shows the mean values of the grating constant along the corrugated area for a typical sample. The mean value for each local grating constant is based on 35 measurements, which leads to a standard deviation of approx. 10^{-4} μm.

Conclusion

The possibilities of a fiber-optic interferometer for integrated optic applications have been confirmed, where the spatial filters have been substituted by two special monomode fibers. Some of the problems arising in connection with interfering gaussian beams as emitted by the fibers have been solved by calculations. With a developed exposure equipment and a suitable monomode fiber we fabricated first samples of chirped grating areas. Their optical performance was measured statistically by a computerized measurement test set.

Acknowledgements

The financial support of parts of this work by the research center of German Federal Post is gratefully acknowledged. The authors also wish to thank Mr. M. Braas for former investigations.

References

1. Handa,Y. et.al., Appl. Opt.,18,248 (1979)
2. Jacob,J., AEÜ, Band 39, 69 (1985)
3. von Lingelsheim,T., IEE Proc. H, 131, 290 (1984)
4. Unrau,U. and Nietz,R., J. Phys. E, 13, 608(1980)
5. Bartolini,R.A.,Appl.Opt., 13, 129 (1974)
6. Bergmann-Schaefer,Band II, Optik, 7.Auflage,deGruyter,Berlin-New York,(1978)

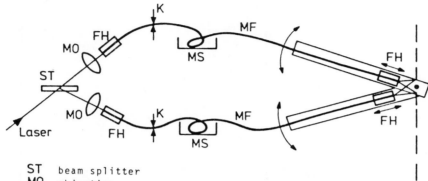

ST	beam splitter
MO	objective
FH	fibre mount
K	fibre clamp
MS	mode stripper
MF	monomode fibre

Figure 1. Configuration of the
fiber-optic interferometer

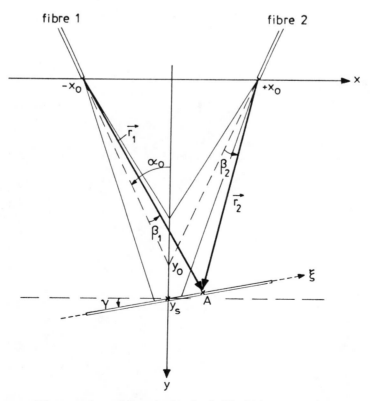

Figure 2. Geometrical definitions

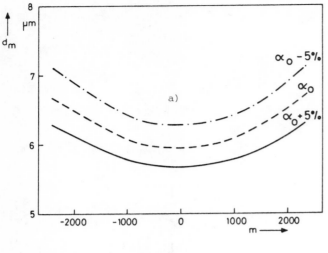

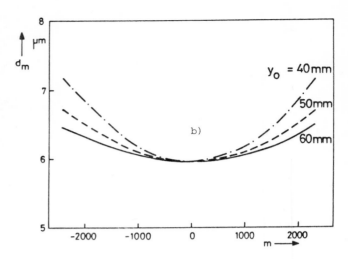

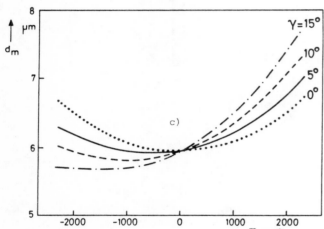

Figure 3. Variable grating constant along
the grating surface

a) with α_O as parameter

b) with y_O as parameter

c) with γ as parameter

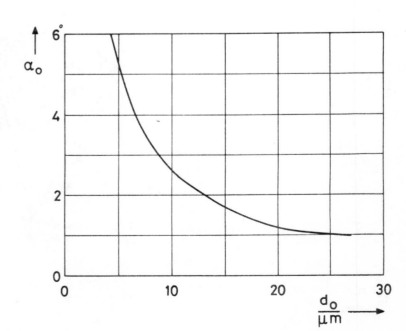

Figure 4. Grating constant in
the center as
function of α_O

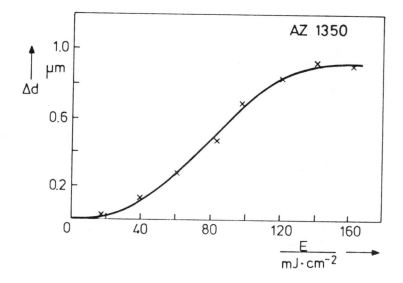

Figure 5. Development characteristic of AZ 1350 resist at 441nm wavelength

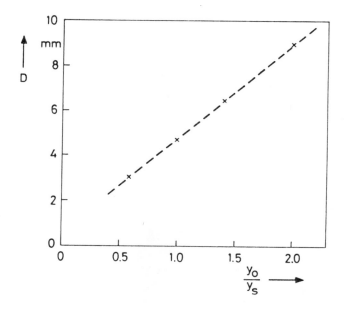

Figure 6. Diameter of the useful interference area as function of relative distance

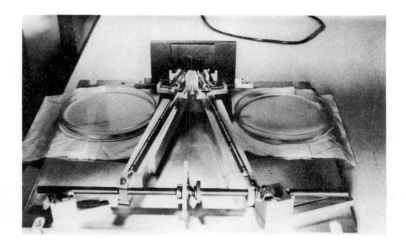

Figure 7. Exposure equipment

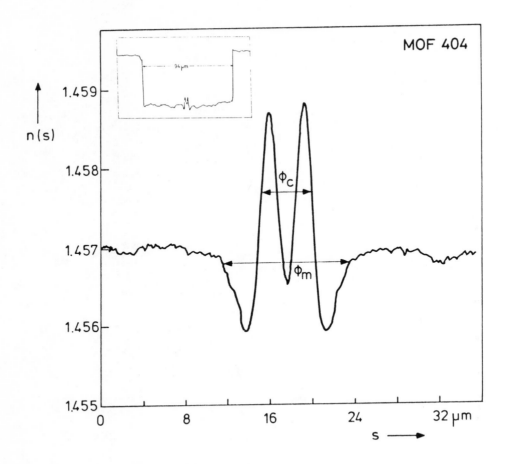

Figure 8. Measured fiber profile

Figure 9. Photoresist grating

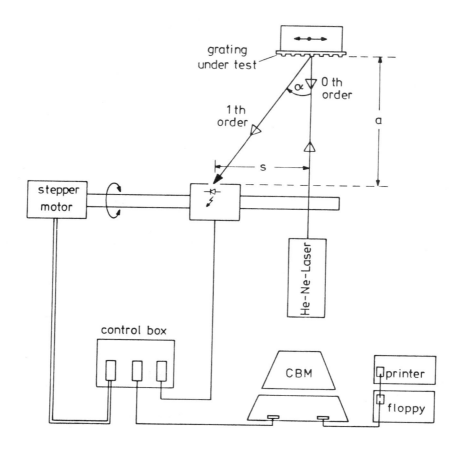

Figure 10. Configuration of the measurement
test set

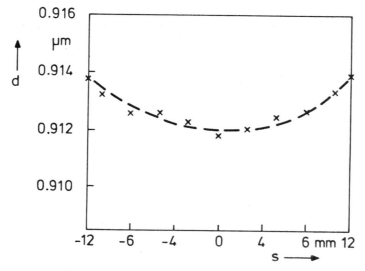

Figure 11. Measured mean values of
the grating constant
(sample HG107/3)

PROGRESS IN HOLOGRAPHIC APPLICATIONS

Volume 600

Session 4

Special Techniques

Chairmen
Gaylord E. Moss
Hughes Aircraft Company, USA
H. J. Caulfield
Aerodyne Research Incorporated, USA

Some problems of computer controlled holography

N.J. Phillips and H. Heyworth

Department of Physics, Loughborough University of Technology
Loughborough, Leics, England

Abstract

A discussion is given of certain aspects of hologram recording using computer control. The computer link is sometimes via direct computation of the fringe pattern of the hologram. This paper discusses the more simplistic and pragmatic use of the computer to control the position of a spot of light thus in effect creating images by point-by-point drawing. It is pointed out that the method has distinct advantages over simultaneous (coherent) recording if certain points of detail are attended to. A method is proposed for the recovery of images of large number of sequentially recorded luminous points.

1. Introduction

Since the earliest origins of modern holography there has been much discussion of the relative merits of the recording of luminous points as a coherent or an incoherent set. Most workers who have made a serious study of the subject are of the opinion that if N holograms are incoherently superimposed in the one recording medium then the efficiency of each is diminished by a factor of $1/N^2$ as compared to the case of a simple recording.

Obviously, when a complex hologram is replayed then the incident light is diffracted into a luminous reconstruction of the elementary points of that image. Sharing of the diffracted light between spatially distributed sources must perforce create a reduction of luminance of any individual point. However, the theoretical analysis is worthy of very careful consideration so that we are absolutely clear about the true physical limitations.

Holography is all about creating a modulation index in a recording medium and then using this modulation to permit recreation of the object defining waves of an initial recording, by interrogations of the hologram with a reference wave. In practice, the technique is fraught with difficulties which stem from the sensitivity and non-linearity of the medium and the basic nature of the interference patterns when we attempt to record. In all non-trivial holographic regimes, the reference to signal ratio is carefully selected to control non-linearity. Too much reference to signal must lead to excessive fog in the recording. This arises because the reference wave cannot be interfered with effectively enough to totally 'stop' it. Thus on balance the 'excess' reference wave simply travels through the medium and sensitises it in a non-informative way. We shall look at this problem in more detail in the next section.

In this paper we shall explore again the fundamental differences between coherent and incoherent superimposed recordings of the image of a luminous point. Certain obvious arguments emerge but our interpretation of the theory is seen to lead to gross differences of approach according to how we accept the theoretical conclusions. We shall see that the elimination of fogging light is of primary concern but the ability to achieve this goal depends critically on the achievement of a recording method which is essentially free from non-linearity. We believe that this freedom from non-linearity can be attained in certain forms of recording with the silver halides and we shall outline an experimental regime with which to exploit the ideas.

We structure this paper in the form of a mathematical discussion of the recording process followed by a discussion of significant experimental recording regimes and their merits. We conclude by offering a short discussion of the work of other contributors to this somewhat neglected field of holographic effort.

2. Theoretical consideration of the recording of a set of luminous points using the holographic method

Let us suppose that we attempt a recording of the interference of a planar reference wave with a spherical wave from a point source. The geometry of the problem is seen overleaf.

We can structure the mathematical theory of interference with varying degrees of accuracy. It is customary to ignore the problems created by polarisation, but in practice these problems cannot be ignored in a condition of minimised fog level. Strictly the simplest of the problems we consider is to treat our interfering waves as polarised in or

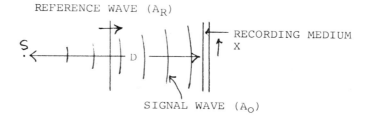

Figure 1: Model for
interference process

out of the plane of the paper and furthermore to ignore the variation of intensity of the
signal wave at the recording page of the hologram.

Let us represent the reference by the amplitude A_R and the signal by the complex
amplitude factor

$$A_S = A_O \left[\exp (ikx^2/2D) \right] = A_O \exp (i\phi) \tag{1}$$

Consider first the incoherent recording of a set of equal amplitude (A_O) elementary
waves of this form so that the total amplitude in the medium can be written in the form

$$A_R + A_O \exp (i\phi_j) \tag{2}$$

for each of N recordings. The recorded intensity becomes

$$I = \sum_{j=1}^{N} \left[A_R + A_O \exp (i\phi_j) \right] \left[A_R + A_O \exp (-i\phi_j) \right] \tag{3}$$

Here A_R will be matched to each of the A_S.

We can look at the intensity in various ways. For example, it is customary to write it
in the form

$$I = \Sigma A_R^2 + \Sigma A_R A_O \exp (-i\phi_j)$$
$$+ \Sigma A_R A_O \exp (+i\phi_j)$$
$$+ \Sigma A_O^2 \tag{4}$$

The complex terms are usually considered in relation to image recovery. They are
proportional to A_R and A_O and hence in a linear system of recording they are directly and
simply interrogated to recreate the signal wave and its complex conjugate respectively.
If all N recordings are of the same amplitude, A_O and A_R is common to all recordings, then

$$I = NA_R^2 + NA_O^2 + 2A_R A_O \sum_{j=1}^{N} \cos (\phi_j) \tag{5}$$

For each term involving ϕ_j we can consider the contribution to the total intensity in the
form

$$I_j = A_R^2 + A_O^2 + 2A_R A_O \cos (\phi_j) \tag{6}$$

We customarily regard the 'modulation index' as the ratio of the fluctuation amplitude
coefficient $2A_R A_O$ to the D.C. level $A_R^2 + A_O^2$. Invariably, due to non-linear problems, we
choose

$$A_R >> A_O$$

This in fact constrains the modulation index. If we write (6) in the form

$$I_j = \underbrace{A_R^2 + A_O^2 - 2A_R A_O}_{\text{D.C. level}} + \underbrace{2A_R A_O \left[1 + \cos (\phi_j) \right]}_{\text{Perfect pattern}} \tag{7}$$

then we have a mixture of D.C. level and a 'perfect pattern' (intensity cannot be negative)
corresponding to the recorded information. This form of the expression is considerably
more instructive than (6), because it also tells us that the D.C. term is of the form

$$I_{jD.C.} = A_R{}^2 + A_O{}^2 - 2A_R A_O = (A_R - A_O)^2 \tag{8}$$

Thus $I_{jD.C.}$ measures the 'catchment' of the signal wave by the reference wave. Imperfect __amplitude__ balance simply creates a __travelling__ or __fogging__ wave situation.

Incoherent recording of the N points thus requires careful balancing in the individual recording events to ensure the minimisation of the expression $(A_R - A_O)^2$. In principle, and to this elementary level of approximation, all points can be recorded without fog and hence with no D.C. bias.

The coherent case of recording may be summarised by the intensity

$$I = \left[A_R + \sum_{j=1}^{N} A_O e^{i\phi_j} \right] \left[A_R + \sum_{j=1}^{N} A_O e^{-i\phi_j} \right] \tag{9}$$

Here the reference intensity $A_R{}^2$ is matched to the summation of signal intensities. If we expand out the expression, we can write it in the form below

$$I = A_R{}^2 + 2A_R A_O \sum_{j=1}^{N} \cos(\phi_j) + A_O{}^2 \sum_{j=1}^{N} \sum_{k=1}^{N} e^{i\phi_j - i\phi_k} \tag{10}$$

$$= A_R{}^2 - 2N A_R A_O + 2A_R A_O \sum_{j=1}^{N} \left[1 + \cos(\phi_j) \right] \tag{11}$$

$$+ N A_O{}^2 + 2 \sum_{j \neq k} \sum A_O{}^2 \cos(\phi_j - \phi_k)$$

There are $N(N-1)/2$ terms in the second summation thus we may write

$$I = A_R{}^2 - 2N A_R A_O + 2A_R A_O \sum_{j=1}^{N} \left[1 + \cos(\phi_j) \right] + N A_O{}^2 - N(N - 1)A_O{}^2 \tag{12}$$

$$+ A_O{}^2 \sum_{j \neq k} \sum \left[1 + \cos(\phi_j - \phi_k) \right]$$

The last term in the expression represents the intermodulation pattern as a 'perfect recording' and the preceeding sum a set of 'perfect patterns' of recording of the information.

Obviously, the importance of the last term can be controlled by the ratio A_R/A_O and in principle the intermodulation can be ignored if the beam ratio is large enough. However, it is apparent that the D.C. level cannot be made to vanish as in the coherent case. Either this intermodulation is ignored (high beam ratio) or is perfectly recorded in which case the hologram is not simply replayable to regenerate only the object waves. We could in principle balance out the D.C. level by making

$$A_R{}^2 - 2N A_R A_O + N A_O{}^2 - N(N - 1)A_O{}^2 = 0 \tag{13}$$

The peculiar structure of this expression is simply due to the fact that the intensity due to N __incoherent__ amplitudes is proportional to $N A_O{}^2$ but is proportional to $N^2 A_O{}^2$ for the coherent case. For large N then the equation (13) yields the solution

$$A_R \simeq N(1 + \sqrt{2})A_O \tag{14}$$

or $A_R{}^2 \propto N^2 A_O{}^2$ so that __coherent__ effects dominate.

The problem which faces us with coherent recording is that elimination of the intermodulation is at the expense of increased fog or D.C. level. This problem is clearly insuperable. The option of recording the __intermodulation__ and the __image patterns__ perfectly is clearly not physically permissible.

We have not yet considered the overall exposure and clearly comparison between the two cases (coherent or incoherent recording) can only be clarified if the exposure problem is outlined. In our experience it has become clear that the correct view of this aspect of the work is actually very subtle. Thus it does not suffice to simply divide the dynamic range of the medium by N the number of recorded points in the case of incoherent overlay. The question of degree of amplification by development arises and we do have this under our control. In our experiments, we have already observed that reduced amplification can be achieved by control of chemistry and if the image is relatively weak then it can be recovered at the stage of phase conjugation.

We conclude finally that there is a strong case for recording the point patterns sequentially so as to avoid the intermodulation and hence permitting the achievement of low fog level. The experimental difficulties are numerous and will emerge in our subsequent discussion.

3. The role of silver halide recording in the context of incoherent outlay of elemental recordings

Feeble overlayed recordings are hardly the province of regimes utilising insensitive recording material. The silver halides offer extreme advantages in this context because they are developable from very weak exposures. Their failing comes in the form of subtle reciprocity failure, a problem dealt with in a detailed paper by Johnson et al[1]. Much confusion exists as to what to do with silver halide material, both at the development stage and in the after-development process. Intrinsic non-linearity of processing can occur when high contrast development is employed.

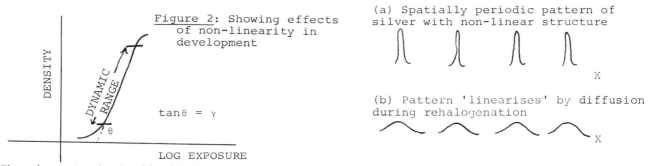

Figure 2: Showing effects of non-linearity in development

$\tan\theta = \gamma$

(a) Spatially periodic pattern of silver with non-linear structure

(b) Pattern 'linearises' by diffusion during rehalogenation

The characteristically high γ achieved when Lippmann emulsions are developed appropriately implies non-linear recording and processing problem with all silver halide materials.

Work within our laboratory in Loughborough has shown that the effect of high contrast in development can be counteracted by a bleach process that modulates the hologram by diffusion transfer. This step is crucially important because as we have discussed earlier any non-linearity can only be counteracted by high beam ratio and hence it must demand a fogging content in the recording light.

Extensive tests have shown that only one method of processing leads to low levels of distortion of the recording of the interference pattern. This method consists of developing the image and following that step by an aqueous rehalogenating bleach. What happens is that silver ion transfers during the bleach and the molecular rearrangement created produces the necessary hologram modulation. The method was first published by one of the authors (N J Phillips and students[2]) and publicised worldwide by Agfa-Gevaert in the method of production of reflection holograms using an Argon laser.

We have shown that Lippmann layers produced by the above technique can be fully modulated yielding reflectances of near 100%. By comparison crude methods of modulation involving fixing or solvent bleaching are unable to approach these results. Theoretical analysis has shown that it is the inherent non-linearity of 'force-majeur' modulation methods that causes a loss of diffraction efficiency into the important first order.

In preliminary experiments, images with some 5000 incoherent superimposed points have been clearly discernible.

4. Image intensification in practical recording systems

Holography is actually a method of recording analogous to electronic phase-sensitive detection. The reference interferes with the signal so long as the wavelengths match. Furthermore, the interference of a 'weak' signal wave with an equally weak reference wave produces strong interference. In practice, of course, such weak wavefronts may require apparatus of great stability. In principle, however, weak, almost imperceptible wavefronts should be recoverable by the method of holographic recording.

Work in these laboratories has outlined several significant methods of noise reduction in holograms and we have successfully exploited these in experiments involving phase conjugation. Even if a 'master' image created in the initial incoherent overlay is weak, we can regenerate it by phase conjugation with a weak reference wave.

5. Necessary ingredients of a successful recording regime for incoherent overlay of point images

The ground rules are now clearly in view. Intermodulation effects have to be avoided as they must perforce increase the fog level. Incoherent overlay with minimal fog is only possible in the case of true point sources (single optical mode). To date, our crude experiments have been performed using a galvanometer scanning system and the creation of the points by illumination of the back of a diffuser plate.

Not surprisingly, the diffuser system shows the problems created by the speckle field (i.e. due to the intermodulation of many optical modes).

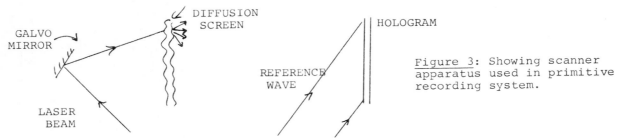

Figure 3: Showing scanner apparatus used in primitive recording system.

The build-up of noise was noticeable after some 500 points were recorded.

Our new system employs a single mode optical fibre system attached to an x,y,z translation stage.

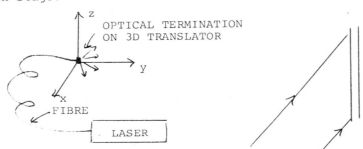

Figure 4: Refined recording system uses single mode non-depolarising optical fibre on three dimensional positioner.

With this method, all intermodulation effects are eliminated. Results from this system are to be reported shortly. The second phase of our method employs simple phase conjugation of one hologram into another.

6. A short and mildly comprehensive guide to some of the significant papers on the subject

We have already mentioned the work of Johnson et al[1] and their discussion of the important problem of what they call 'holographic reciprocity law failure'. This paper is of great importance as it ingeniously describes the unwanted interaction between subsequent exposures of the holographic medium. Summarising such a detailed paper is difficult but suffice it to say that they show that photo-electrons created by one exposure but which do not in effect create a developable grain can carry over from one exposure to the next. When second exposure occurs then grains which were not developable at the first exposure can become developable at the second. Thus the previous exposure can be 'boosted' by the second and hence the optical density of the developed hologram is not truly a set of independent density effects. These authors point out that modification of one exposure pattern by previous or subsequent exposures could for instance lead to inaccurate interpretation of medical photographic overlays used in 3D viewing systems. Putting this paper out of historical order is deliberate as it offers more education concerning the formation of the holographic image than probably any other in the field.

Historically, we find an elementary attempt at point by point drawing on the paper by Spitz and Werts[3] which discusses the drawing of the image of a cube in three dimensions.

The holographic synthesis of computer generated holograms was considered by Stroke et al[4]. Claimed syntheses include holograms of objects with more than one thousand object points.

The paper by LaMacchia and White[5] discusses the use of a coded reference beam system. Each hologram was formed with a uniquely coded reference beam allowing reconstruction of only one of the superimposed holograms while the unaddressed holograms contributed incoherent noise. For a one thousand exposure hologram the observed signal to noise ratio for any one hologram was 10dB.

La Macchia and Vincelette[6] discuss the efficiency of multiple exposure and single exposure holograms and conclude that the efficiency for M holograms is more probably $\alpha 1/M$ than the usual $1/M^2$ law. Experimental validation of this conclusion is offered.

Kozma and Massey[7] discuss a novel time modulation technique in one path of an interferometer to assist in removal of the D.C. bias problem. The holograms are essentially of 2D objects but the results are convincing, though probably not generalisable to 3D.

In the paper by Spasov et al[8] the $1/N^2$ law is taken as correct. Some experimental verification is described by reference to holograms formed in unbleached plates with colloidal development techniques.

Landry et al[9] consider some forms of bleach chemistry for Agfa 10E75 material and discuss diffraction efficiencies for single and multiple exposure recordings. These results are interesting but though the detail of their work is considerable, the results are not encouraging probably due to rather primitive chemical techniques employed.

Rhodes[10] discusses the bias problem and a novel method of partial hologram recording to improve the signal to noise ratio. This is more a conceptual paper than a demonstration, but nonetheless is a tidy and very competent discussion of the difficulties.

Caulfield et al[11] discuss the bias problem and quote results showing an image of over 4000 successive exposures. Caulfield[12] then goes on to resurrect the problem in an important paper discussing the merits of partial illumination of the hologram by the reference beam and reporting a novel point movement procedure to speed up the recording process.

If we summarise these papers, we see varying degrees of success with this problem but a variable approach to both the theoretical and the experimental aspects. The acceptance of the $1/N^2$ law is more an act of faith than the result of precise and well reasoned argument. This law will certainly apply in the case where the beam ratio is used to induce linearity of the reconstruction process. However, as we have pointed out here, this is not the only regime of importance.

It is our considered view that the subject is still wide open and that approaches such as those of Caulfield may make major advances.

In conclusion, we note that silver halide recording is much more complex than was initially thought to be the case and the work of Johnson et al[1] has to be a subject of major preoccupation. However, the theoretical forms discussed vary from one approach to another and most show some departure from total physical or analytical rigour. Perhaps another look at this problem will pay big dividends.

7. Summary

We have presented cogent arguments supporting the possibility of the incoherent overlay of point image recordings. The ideas are not new but they represent another look at an old story. Our view of the mathematics and the physics must be associated with physically realisable systems. We have seen that increasingly the reference to signal ratio is a palliative but it exacerbates the fundamental problem of fog level.

As a back-up to the primary recording of weak images, we always have recourse to the phase sensitive detection aspect of holography. What matters is our ability to dump the noise from the master hologram.

Great promise is shown by our early experiments but future work will be supported by the new low noise Ilford recording materials thus considerable improvements are to be expected. A discussion of the performance of our complete system will be reported in the near future.

Acknowledgements

This work has been made possible by support from the Central Electricity Generating Board and ICI plc in England, together with the resources of Loughborough University of Technology.

References

1. Johnson, K.M., Hesselink, L. and Goodman, J.W., Applied Optics, Vol 123, No 2, 1984.
2. Phillips, N.J., Ward, A.A., Cullen, R. and Porter, D., Phot. Sci. and Eng., Vol 24,

No 2, 1980.

3. Spitz, E. and Werts, A., Comptes Rendues Acad. Sci. Paris, Vol 262, March 1966.
4. Stroke, G.W., Westervelt, F.H. and Zech, R.G., I.E.E.E. Proc. 109, 55, 1967.
5. LaMacchia, J.T. and White, D.L., Applied Optics, Vol 17, No 1, 91-94, 1968.
6. LaMacchia, J.T. and Vincelette, C.J., Applied Optics, Vol 17, No 9, 1857-1858, 1968.
7. Kozma, A. and Massey, N., Applied Optics, Vol 18, No 2, 393-397, 1969.
8. Spasov, G.A., S"imov, K. and S"ynov, S., Autometriya (USSR), 3, 93-95, 1981.
9. Landry, M.J., Phipps, G.S. and Robertson, C.E., Applied Optics, Vol 17, No 11, 1764-1770, 1978.
10. Rhodes, W.T., Proc. S.P.I.E. Inst. Soc. Opt. Eng., 437, 90-95, 1983.
11. Caulfield, H.J., Lu, S. and Harris, J.L., Applied Optics 58, 1003-1004, 1967.
12. Caulfield, H.J., Proc. S.P.I.E., Vol 402, 114-118, 1983.

Aspects of the copying of holograms using incoherent light

N J Phillips (1) and D Martens (2)

(1) Department of Physics, University of Technology, Loughborough, Leics, LE11 3TU, U.K.
(2) Department of Applied Physics, Twente University of Technology, Twente, The Netherlands

Abstract

Copying of holograms using laser light in a contact situation is a commonplace technique. This paper discusses the use of simplistic incoherent light sources and filters to achieve the same result. Results are reported of test experiments which show that existing holographic recording emulsions are barely adequate in structure and performance. Theoretical criteria are reported which offer guidance for the optimised use of the recording media.

1. Introduction

In recent papers, the writer and students have discussed experimental and theoretical aspects of the formation of reflective Lippmann layers using partially coherent light (Phillips, Heyworth and Harel[1]; Phillips and van der Werf[2]). This work consisted of revisiting the work of Lippmann to assess the true optical and physico-chemical limitations of the recording of reflection layers by photography rather than holography.

What we found was that surprisingly high levels of reflectance could be induced in silver halide layers with results approaching those only previously achieved with dichromated gelatin (D.C.G.). To date, we have not observed modulation mechanisms which quite compare with those in D.C.G. in terms of order of magnitude of phase shift induced. It is, for example, well known that D.C.G. can be modulated so heavily that broadband reflective effects can be achieved without great difficulty. With the silver halides, there has been no equivalent observation although certain methods of development of silver halide layers can produce very high reflectances accompanied by broadband effects, but with unacceptable grain scatter and dichroic fog.

Our work on the mechanisms of modulation and processing in Lippmann layers was prompted amongst other reasons by a desire to establish whether one could in fact create holograms by using simplistic weakly coherent sources of light.

A detailed discussion[1] of the fundamentals of hologram recording revealed the somewhat obvious difficulties posed by random phase variation during the recording of fringes in the Lippmann layer. Though we claimed nothing new in terms of this discussion, it became possible to see that the main advantage of Lippmann's mirrored recording regime for reflectors simply depended on the insensitivity of the method to the absolute phase of the recording light.

All three-dimensionally encoded interference structures of the holographic type have a common property. They have built in to them interference fringes which are sympathetic to both a signal wave and what we usually call a reference wave. Whether the signal wave or the reference wave is made dominant is a matter of choice. For most simplistic display holograms the intensity of the reference wave is made dominant so as to ensure linearity of the recording process. However, 'robotics vision' might require holograms in which the 'signal' wave regenerates the reference wave as a method of position sensing.

The sympathy of the fringes to two or more different types of wavefront can only be achieved if the relative phase of the wavefronts in any locality in the recording medium is held constant. For this reason holograms can usually only be made in light of organised phase (coherent light). Any relaxation of the stringent control of coherence usually results in problems, except when say the simplistic Lippmann reflector is to be fabricated or perhaps when certain forms of optically simplistic white light interferometers are used to create fringes. In general, when informative recordings are made by the technique of holography, then a laser has to be used in the recording process. The laser offers advantages of both extremes of spatial and temporal coherence in the recording process though in fact this very excellence can lead to problems of speckle and lack of image definition in the use of holograms to create images of three-dimensional objects.

Relaxation of spatial coherence of the recording light is often difficult to achieve without certain concommitant penalties but the most severe restriction probably relates to attempted relaxation of temporal coherence as we shall see.

We have undertaken simple experiments to achieve the copying of both relief image holograms and Lippmann volume holograms using the light from a Sodium discharge source and subsequently light from a tungsten-halogen lamp with a high quality single spectral line Sodium filter placed in front of the lamp. We shall outline some of our findings below together with a discussion of the experimental regimes.

2. Theoretical discussion of the interference of partially coherent light in the formation of Lippmann layers

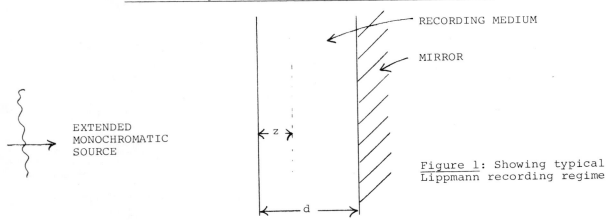

Figure 1: Showing typical Lippmann recording regime

In[1], we discussed the formation of fringes in a Lippmann layer with a range of wavelengths, $\lambda_1 \rightarrow \lambda_2$, or wavenumbers $k_1 \rightarrow k_2$. In an equal energy recording the intensity of light in the recording medium can be seen to be (here λ_1, λ_2, k_1, k_2 are referred to the recording media)

$$I = 2A^2(k_2-k_1) \left[1 - \cos\left[(k_2+k_1)(z-d)\right] \sin c \left[(k_2-k_1)(z-d)\right]\right] \qquad (1)$$

where A is the amplitude of the light arriving from the left of the recording medium and $\sin c\ x = \sin x/x$. We called this the 'blur model' because it simply reflects the fact that as the range of wavelengths $(k_2 - k_1)$ increase then the spatial range over which high contrast fringes are observed diminishes; beyond a certain point in the layer, the pattern is blurred.

We might then set a figure of merit based upon the criterion $\sin c \left[(k_2 - k_1)d\right] > 96\%$ say. This would in turn imply that fringes are clearly visible throughout the recording layer if

$$|k_2 - k_1|d < 0.5 \qquad (2)$$

What we proposed was that in the absence of such a demand, we might realistically consider the practical experience with heavily modulated Lippmann layers, suggesting that some six Lippmann planes might be enough to create an efficient albeit not too selective recording layer.

The first zero of the sin c function is reached when

$$\sin c \left[(k_2 - k_1)(z - d)\right] = 0 \qquad (3)$$

i.e. when

$$(z - d)(k_2 - k_1) = \pi \qquad (4)$$

Suppose that we take a mid-spectrum yellow-green wavelength at say 550nm in a gelatin layer whose refractive index $n \simeq 1.54$ say, then six Lippmann planes implies a layer of thickness of the order of $1\mu m$. From equation (4), we see that a bandwidth limitation for the recording light is set by the relation

$$\delta = \frac{\lambda_{1a}\lambda_{2a}}{2n\Delta\lambda}$$

where δ is the thickness of the zone of high contrast fringes in the emulsion and $\Delta\lambda = \lambda_{2a} - \lambda_{1a}$. Setting $\delta = 1\mu$, $\lambda_{1a} \simeq \lambda_{2a} \simeq 550$nm, we have

$$\Delta\lambda \simeq 0.1\mu$$

In practice, filters which are monochromatically transmissive are available with a bandwidth $\Delta\lambda \simeq 0.02\mu$ so that such filters are eminently suitable for the recording process when used in conjunction with a small white source such as a tungsten halogen bulb.

In the recording of simplistic Lippmann reflectors then, the source size is not much of a problem either. We undertook[2] recordings with F numbers as low as f2.

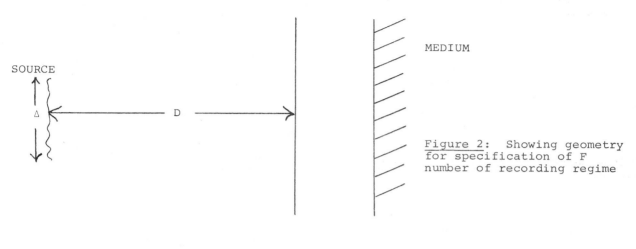

Figure 2: Showing geometry for specification of F number of recording regime

$$F \text{ number} = \frac{D}{\Delta}$$

3. Preliminary experimental results of recording of Lippmann layers and contact copied holograms with filtered natural light

It was relatively easy to create nearly perfect Lippmann reflectances with Sodium discharge light. Here we have $\Delta\lambda = 0.0006\mu$, so that despite its doublet structure Sodium light is nearly as good as a laser for the job. We compared these perfected results with those created using a narrow band 'Sodium' filter ($\Delta\lambda \simeq 0.02\mu$) and found that in the simplistic non-holographic case, then reflectances were approximately equal to those created with the Sodium discharge lamp.

The major area of problem lay with our ability to create good contact between the recording medium and the mirror behind it. We had established that mirrors were best made of metallised mylar, but that dust or surface irregularities due to filler in the mylar were a major problem.

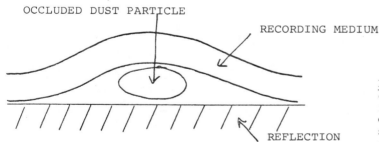

Figure 3: 'Lift-off' of contacted film layer may cause fringes of **unequal** thickness or low efficiency due to separation of recording layer from mirror.

Areas of poor contact displayed severe cosmetic fringe difficulties which were nowhere near as predominant in the case of Sodium discharge recording.

Evidently, contact imaging, however simple, requires scrupulous cleanliness of the interface between the recording medium and the reflective surface underneath.

We also found that delays between application of the contacting fluid and recording could be excessive (c. 0.5hr) but further work established that mild warming in a drying cabinet (T < 30ºC) greatly speeded the process of excess contact fluid removal.

Contact copying of holograms certainly works with this methodology but if the master surface is that of a Lippmann hologram then of course we need to match wavelengths of recording light to the holographic structure in the master. Some compensation for this problem can be achieved by angling the reference, but only at the expense of image astigmatism.

From the underlying principles, we expected that the dead space in the gelatin film which is created by the pressure relief layer would present a major problem in the case of filtered natural light.

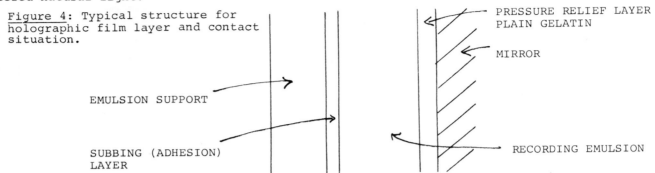

Figure 4: Typical structure for holographic film layer and contact situation.

EMULSION SUPPORT

SUBBING (ADHESION) LAYER

PRESSURE RELIEF LAYER
PLAIN GELATIN

MIRROR

RECORDING EMULSION

This pressure relief layer is normally applied during coating of the film to inhibit the sensitization of surface grains in the emulsion by pressure

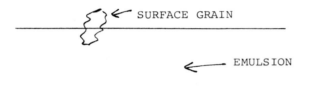

SURFACE GRAIN

EMULSION

Figure 5: Showing 'large' grain near surface of photographic emulsion.

This problem can be very severe in the case of X-ray emulsions and can cause false diagnosis in critical X-ray analysis of human physical defects. By coating the emulsion surface with a thin layer of plain gelatin, the problem is largely alleviated. However, tests with holographic emulsions where the grain size is much smaller (c. 0.03μm) have shown little tendency for the lack of the pressure relief layer to be a problem. It is pointed out however that in the large-scale manufacture of films, then it is all too easy to scratch the emulsion surface. The plain gelatin layer if scratched is essentially 'self healing'. Whether such a coating-free emulsion is practical as far as manufacture is concerned remains to be seen.

4. Summary

We have shown that effective contact copying of holographic surfaces can be achieved using our published method and some care in the choice of filtered natural light.

Advances in emulsion technology have strongly suggested that this method of replication of holograms will become an important commercial technique in the future.

The problems posed by the requirement of intimate contact of the copy and the master surface can be relieved by firstly cleanliness and secondly by removal of the pressure relief layer on the film.

Our evidence to date is that the ability of filtered natural light to 'contact copy' Lippmann holograms or create Lippmann reflectors is just as good as that of the Sodium discharge. Exciting developments in silver halide emulsion technology make this area of study of great interest in the future.

Acknowledgements

Miss Martens' work was performed during a summer stay at Loughborough University as part of her student training at Twente.

References

1. Phillips, N.J., Heyworth, H. and Hare, T., J. Phot. Sci. 32, No.5, 158-169, 1984.
2. Phillips, N.J. and van der Werf, R.A.J., J. Phot. Sci. 33, No.1, 22-28, 1985.

Holography of very far objects

H. Royer

Institut Franco-allemand de Recherches (ISL)
68301 Saint-Louis, France

Abstract

We describe a high-luminosity holographic system which allows the recording of large volumes at a long distance. A high-resolution image is reconstructed, which allows accurate measurements to be achieved in the object. The arrangement is adapted to double-exposure recording with two separate references. An application to ballistics is presented .

Introduction

The increasing interest taken in holography by scientists in many areas has given rise to new applications in various domains. However, all these applications have common limits: the maximum volume and the maximum object-to-hologram distance are imposed by the energy and by the coherence length of the light source. Moreover the resolution in the image is limited by the hologram size.

Large scenes have already been recorded at few meters[1] but they were only intended to visual observation. A certain number of physical studies require that the objects remain far from the optical system (dangerous phenomena) but the resolution should be high enough to allow accurate measurements in the 3-dimensional image. The use of holography sets particular problems in this case.

Problems related to the object distance

If a hologram is recorded with the help of a lensless system, the energy W of the laser pulse is related to the plate sensitivity σ and to the object distance D by:

$$\sigma = 3 \; KW/D^2 \qquad\qquad (1)$$

K is the angular reflectivity of the object ($K = 1/2 \; \pi \; sr^{-1}$ for a perfect diffuser). Thus the recording of a scene at 10 meters with a standard holographic plate ($\sigma = 2 \; \mu J/cm^2$) may require an energy of few tens of joules. On the other hand, the resolution obtained in these conditions with a 100 cm^2 plate would not exceed 7 lines/mm at this distance.

To fulfil the coherence requirements of the light source, the optical path variations corresponding to the different parts of the object scene must remain smaller than its coherence length (one or two meters). These variations are directly depending on the scene depth if a normal front illumination is used.

Use of an imaging lens

The perception of the details as well as of the relief in the object is proportional to the angular aperture of the object beam. To compensate the increase of the object distance while keeping standard-size plates, it is necessary to introduce a large aperture lens which images the scene near the hologram[2]. This gives rise to a difficulty: the magnification of the primary image is very low (about 1:20 for a distance of 10 meters). Thus a detail of 100 μm in the object corresponds to few microns in the image and the hologram resolution must be as high as to reconstruct it.

As a consequence it is important to reduce the aberrations generated by an eventual change of wavelength[3] due to the change of laser between the recording and the reconstruction. For this reason we have compared theoretically and experimentally three types of recording arrangements:
a) the object beam is normal to the plate while the reference arrives at 45°,
b) the reference is normal to the plate and the object beam arrives at 45°,
c) the two beams arrive symetrically at 45°.

The first arrangement has shown itself the best and indeed the only acceptable for a wavelength change of 10% (ruby → He-Ne lasers).

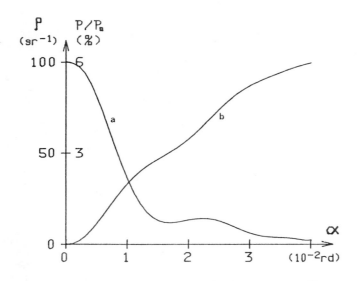

Figure 1. a) Diffusion factor of the retroreflector as a
function of the angle α
b) Relative energy collected by a lens of aperture 2α centered on the incident beam

Object field illumination

Equation (1) shows that it is possible to improve the system by modifying the value of K. Covering the object with bright paint only suits if it has large dimensions. If the object is composed of small elements scattered in the view field, it is better to illuminate it from the rear. For this purpose we have used retroreflecting tape to wallpaper the scene background. This technique has proved efficient in bubble-chamber visualization experiments[4].

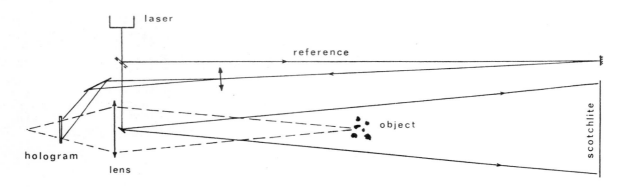

Figure 2. Schematic diagram of the recording set-up

Compared to a perfect diffuser, the retroreflector provides a gain of 600 when its position is optimized, i.e. when the imaging lens is just covered by its diffusion peak (fig.1).

a) In addition to the gain of brightness, this system has other advantages.
In this configuration the optical paths covered by the object rays are practically independent of the scene depth. This means that a very deep field can be recorded with no special requirement for the source coherence.

b) A displacement of the object during the exposure has no other effect than the classical blur. This allows applications to high-speed phenomenon studies.

As a counterpart, the object contours only are visible in the image but this is enough to achieve accurate measurements of its size, shape, position and velocity.

Double-exposure velocimetry

To obtain double-exposure holograms we have used two independent laser cavities. This allows the time interval between the pulses to vary from zero to infinite. The two object beams meet on the diffusing background, then they travel together. The references remain separate and they arrive symmetrically on the plate in order to produce images of same quality.

This system allows the two images to be reconstructed as well simultaneously as separately. The first mode allows a better adjustement of their relative positions while the second mode provides a high contrast for more accurate measurements.

Experimental set-up

For each exposure the light beam coming from the corresponding laser is divided into two parts by a simple prism of small angle. The object wave (80% of the incident energy) is transmitted through the prism. Then a small mirror located before the imaging lens reflects the beam toward the background panel, 15 meters away. The light diffused by the panel illuminates the object field which is located half-way from the lens. Thus when the object is in focus, its shadow on the diffuser is too fuzzy to disturb its image.

The reference wave is reflected on the prism. It covers the same distance as the object beam between the beamsplitter and the hologram, i.e. more than 30 meters. Figure 2 shows a schematic diagram of the arrangement.

Results and conclusion

Various objects have been recorded in our laboratory at a distance of 8 meters. A volume of the other of 1 m³ has been reconstructed with a resolution of about 100 μm. Double-exposure reconstructions have shown the feasibility of velocity measurements at the same distance (fig. 3).

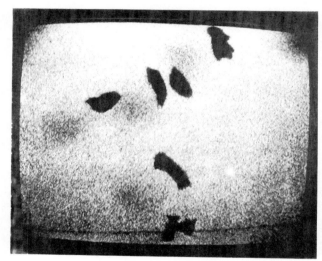 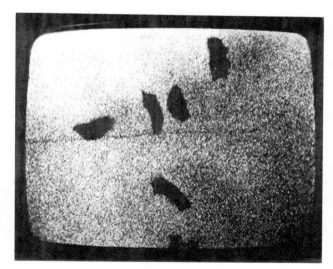

Figure 3. A wire (out of focus) reveals the displacements of the fragments between exposures a) and b). Distance: 8 meters

An application of the method has also been achieved in an outdoor ballistic experiment. Fragments projected at 1800 m/s by a high-energy explosive charge were to be visualized in three dimensions. This gave rise to additional problems related to the presence of daylight as well as to the very intense vibrations and to the air blow generated by the explosion. A 15 mJ monomode ruby laser was used for these experiments. Its coherence length was of the order of 1,5 meter. Figure 4 shows an example of reconstruction achieved in these conditions. The images are focussed respectively at 10 m and 13 m.

The low energy of the laser used for these experiments shows that it is still possible to improve the results by increasing the field of view or the object distance. On the other hand, the method should be useful in the domain of holographic interferometry applied to dangerous objects. For example the behaviour of a working propeller or the distortion of an explosive-charge envelope before the rupture could be studied by this technique.

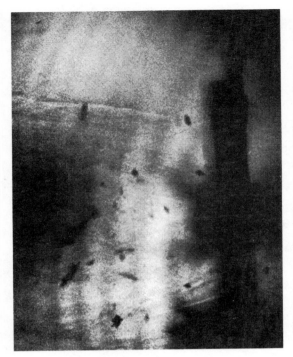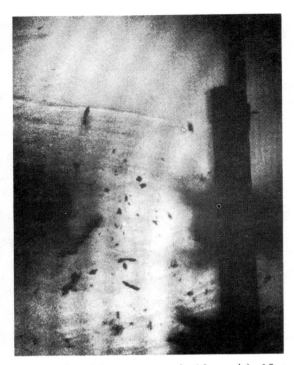

Figure 4.   Fragments impinging a target at 1800 m/s. Distances: a) 10 m; b) 13 m

References

1.   Hirth, A., Vollrath, K., ISL Report RT 13/71 (1971)
2.   Briones, R.A., SPIE 215-112 (1980)
3.   Royer, H., Marquet, M., C.R. Acad. Sc. Paris 260-6051 (1965)
4.   Pouyat, F., BEBC Newsletter (CERN) 18.6 (1981)

Holographic device for analysis of objects inaccessible by direct microscopic technique

J. Surget

Office National d'Etudes et de Recherches Aérospatiales,
BP 72, 92322 Châtillon Cedex, FRANCE.

Abstract

In contrast with ordinary photographic techniques, a three dimensional analysis of transparent or opaque objects can be obtained by holographic technique, with combined properties which are not obtainable simultaneously by classical optics, namely: high resolution, wide field of view, large frontal distance. The last property is very useful in the case of difficult access to the object plane for any reason such as: cumbersome mechanics, safety considerations...

A holographic device has been built for the investigation of the rectilinear discharge propagation on a surface intended to simulate, in the laboratory, the natural leader lightning phenomenon. The apparatus was designed in order to achieve both high temporal and spatial resolution, without neglecting the necessity of a minimum value of forty centimeters for the distance between the set-up and the electric phenomenon (120 kV). No optical component is placed between the object plane and the hologram plate. So, the resolution of the record only depends on the angle substending the holographic plate as measured from the object.

A single exposure is used for the record of a hologram providing the shadowgraphy of the channel (optical phase object). The interferometric examination is also possible by means of the double exposure holographic method.

With just a few minor modifications, the holographic set-up was also used for the study of the structure of a turbulent flame, for the high resolution record of opaque objects and the interferometric examination of their deformations.

The reconstruction, from the holograhic plate, of a high resolution real image at the same size of the object is achieved by means of another especially designed set-up. So, this three dimensional image can be easily observed by means of a microscope, unlike the phenomenon itself which is brief and/or inaccessible.

The two optical devices are described and various examples of applications are given.

Introduction

The observation of an object or luminous phenomenon under high magnification requires an optical system with a wide numerical aperture. The size e_M of the smallest object that can be resolved depends on the aperture angle u of the observation optics (fig. 1a) as determined by the well-known relation:

$$e_M = \frac{0.6\,\lambda}{n\,\sin u}$$

where λ is the wavelength and n is the refractive index of the ambiant medium.

When the observation distance is no more than a few millimeters, as in classical microscopy, u can be given very large values. But when the test conditions make it necessary to place the instrument several hundreds of millimeters from the object, the objective lens diameter must be increased so much, to obtain the same resolving power, that its construction is no longer feasible. Because of this, until recent years it has not been possible to investigate many phenomena that would normally be suitable for microscopic analysis but are physically difficult to approach.

Today, however, holography can serve as a relay between the phenomenon and the observation instrument, thus expanding the limits of microscopy considerably.

In holography the resolving power also depends on the angle of aperture u from the center of the field to the center and edge of the photographic plate H used for the holographic recording. Only those objects diffracting the light that illuminate them inside the perimeter of H can be resolved (fig. 1b). However, it is more easier to have a large photographic plate than a giant microscope objective.

The size e_H of the smallest object resolved is given by the following expression, very similar than the first:

$$e_H = \frac{\lambda}{n\,\sin u}$$

Holography offers several crucial advantages: firstly it does not require the presence of an optical element in the immediate vicinity of the phenomenon being studied; but also it reconciles high resolving power with a wide field, which are contradictory ideas in conventional optics; in last, it provides a three dimensional image.

The method consists of recording a hologram of the object at a distance, under very precise conditions that ensures the desired definition in the image, to be reconstructed afterwards.

After processing, the hologram is illuminated, not to reconstruct the virtual image usually observed through the photographic plate, but in such a way as to set up a real image reconstructed between the plate and the observer. So, this image can be studied by means of a magnifier or a microscope.

The observation is thus in "delayed time" but there are several important advantages, previously mentionned, to off-set this: the object can be both far away and large, the scale of the restituted 3-D image is 1/1, and the resolution may be high.

Therefore, the association of holography and microscopy by this technique has beneficial applications in a variety of fields, such as:

- 3-D recording of aerosol particles which are later measured to find the diameters and space distribution;
- recording elementary particles trajectories in bubble chambers;
- velocity measurement of liquid or gas flow seeded with tracers;
- analysis of explosions or projectile impacts, etc.

For these studies, the "in line" holography is used on account of its simplicity, mainly for the real image reconstruction[1] to [3]. However, a high resolution real image can be also obtained in the case of "off line" holography, if the reference beam used is free from optical aberrations, as demonstrated by the experiments described in this paper.

The holographic image transport technique was used at ONERA in first for the study of the propagation of a gliding spark, simulating an atmospheric leader lightning in the discharge laboratory of Chalais-Meudon[4]: a holographic set-up, specially adapted to the discharge channel visualization and measurement, was built[5], and successfully used[6].

On account of its versatility, the holographic apparatus was then used, with just few minor modifications, for other applications: mainly the high resolution three dimensional image recording of opaque objects and the interferometric examination of their deformations, the measurement and space location of the outline of small objects, and the study of the structure of a turbulent flame.

gliding spark study

The two aims of this study are the measurement of the radius of the channel, and the refractive index of the gas inside it.

As the radius channel varies from 100 to 300 μm depending on the test conditions, a microscope is needed to measured it. However, it was impossible to observe the arc directly in a microscope since the 120,000 V electric potential used for the experiment requires a 400 mm distance for safety. Moreover, for each discharge, the channel has to be examined over a lenght of some 150 mm, which is of course much greater than the microscope field of view.

The briefness to the phenomenon should be mentionned as one final difficulty: the spark propagation speed goes from 1,000 to 2,000 km/s.

Holographic device

The holographic device is shown in figure 2 with its various components arranged on a 1.20 x 0.80 m granite table, 4 cm thick.

Figure 3 shows the apparatus as installed in the discharge laboratory. The dark panel standing in the back is a polished black plexiglass wall, serving as a dielectric. The spark glides over this panel, guided by an electrode vertically fixed on its rear surface[4].

The holographic bench does not touch the plexiglass, but is located 400 mm away as indicated in the optical diagram of the experiment (figure 4).

The laser is not part of the holographic device, but is placed a sufficient distance from the plexiglass panel P raised to the 120,000 V potential. The laser is a pulsed yag with frequency doubled, delivering 220 mJ in 15 ns at the wavelenght 0.532 μm.

The unexpanded laser beam enters the holographic device and is first reflected in a total internal reflection prism P1.

The light reflected by P1 is then divided into two beams (the test beam E and the reference beam R), by a glass plate S inclined at the Brewster's angle. S is bracketed by two in-plane rotating half-waves crystalline plates D1 and D2. This beam splitter, already tested elsewhere[7], provides a way for controlling continuously the ratio of the E and R light intensities. This ratio varies greatly, depending whether transparent or opaque objects are being recorded. So it is important to be able to modify the ratio easily on a test stand that is supposed to be put to several purposes.

The laser beam transmitted by S is reflected by prism P2 in the direction of the afocal lens system L1 and L2. The diameter of the expanding parallel beam emerging from L2 depends on the size of this lens (here 145 mm in diameter).

The test beam E strikes plexiglass panel P at a 12° angle of incidence. P reflects a few percent of the incident light flux in the direction of the photographic plate H used to record the hologram.

The light emission accompanying the electric discharge is much lower than the laser beam in plane H. For this reason, from the optical point of view, the channel can be said to behave like a simple transparent medium (phase object) that the light beam passes through twice, once before and once after its reflection from P.

The photographic plate H is perpendicular to the test beam, to make sure the holographic image undergoes as geometric distorsion as possible when it is reconstructed with a continuous laser emitting at a different wavelength from the pulsed laser used for the recording[2].

No optical components are placed between the object plane P and the photographic plate H, here again to avoid as much as possible the risks of altering the image. The photographic plate is the closest element of the instrument to the object plane, giving the aperture angle u (figure 1b) the maximum value it can obtain considering the set 400 mm safety distance from the object plan.

For the 102 x 127 mm photographic plate format and a 0.532 μm wavelength, expression (2) in the previous section gives a theoretical 3.5 μm value for the smallest object that can be resolved. Such a resolution, over the entire 145 mm field observed at this distance, cannot of course be obtained by conventional photographic technics. In fact, the real holographic resolution is slightly degraded by the ligth wavefront distorsion introduced by the poor optical quality of the photoplate glass.

The reference beam R, reflected by S, follows a path roughly symmetrical to that of the test beam E (figure 4). The two 45° prisms P3 are used to equalize the length of the reference beam path with that of the test beam. The afocal lens system comprising L3 and L4 (145 mm in diameter) expanses the reference beam which is then directed to the photoplate H by the plane mirror M placed near the object plane P.

Reconstruction device. The optical diagram for the reconstruction device is given in figure 5. The light source is a C.W. laser for comfortable observation of the reconstructed image. Its wavelength must be as closed as possible to the one used for recording (λ = 0.532 μm) to minimize both the change in magnification and any geometric distorsion that may occur due to the change of wavelength. In the present case, an argon ion laser is used, emitting at λ = 0.514 μm. The afocal device, comprising the same lenses L3 and L4 as the holographic recording bench (figure 4) also produces a reference beam of parallel light rays.

The use of reference source at infinity for object recording and image reconstruction is advantageous: the processed hologram produces one virtual image and one real image, at the same magnification (unity), placed symmetrically with it. One or the other image is observed by reversing the direction of propagation of the light with respect to the hologram[8]. This reversal is particularly easy to make when the reference beam is made up of parallel rays, because the plate H has simply to be turned around. It is much less convenient when the reference beam used for recording is a divergent cone, as is commonly the case, because beams having exactly the same angle, but respectively divergent and convergent, are then needed to observe the reconstructed virtual and real images.

The rotating plate holder P₁ of the reconstruction device (figure 5) makes it easy to observe the virtual or the real holographic image:

- figure 5a: when the processed photoplate H is illuminated the same way as during exposure (emulsion facing the incident beam) the virtual image P' is observed through H at the place corresponding to the plan P containing the phenomenon under study (figure 4);
- figure 5b: by turning H of 180°, which comes down to reversing the direction of light propagation, the reconstructed real image P' appears between the photoplate and the observer. So, this image can be easily observed and recorded.

Experiments and results. Systematic tests were performed with different delays after the spark ignition.

Two holographic methods were used to visualize the discharge channel:
- a single exposure of the photoplate H (figure 4) for the recording of a hologram providing the shadowgraph of the phenomenon;
- a double exposure of H, for obtaining its interferogram; the first exposure before the start of the spark, and the second with a delay ΔT after crossing of the spark to the field apparatus.

In fact, the interferometric method was mainly used. Figure 6 shows four examples of finite fringe interferograms obtained by this technique for several values of ΔT.

The radius of the channel and the shift of the refractive index inside it are given by the deformation of the original straight pattern;

The hologram data processing leads to the knowledge of the temporal channel radius increasing and refractive index variation[6].

Opaque objects recording

A minor modification of the device makes it possible to record opaque objects (figure 7). It is just necessary to put the object A in place of the plexiglass panel P in the original set-up (figure 4). The light from the test beam scattered by A interferes with the light from the reference beam to form the hologram recorded by the photoplate H.

Only is possible the recording of objects comprising into the coherence lenght of the laser. The reconstruction device is unchanged (figure 5).

Figure 8 shows three reconstructed images of a 30 mm disk photographed by receiving it on a photographic emulsion (without objective). This figure demonstrates the effect that any defects in L4 lenses in either the recording or reconstruction systems (figures 5 and 7) may have on the quality of the reconstructed image.

The degree of ressemblance of the virtual image with the object only depends on the similitude of the two reference beams of the devices used for recording and reconstruction. In others words, any aberrations in these two beams are of little importance as long as the beams are identical. In contrary, to reconstruct the real image, the reference beam must be free from any aberrations, and must just consist of perfectly parallel rays.

In effect, if the reference beams used for recording and reconstruction have, for example, the same small divergence defect, the incidence defect is doubled by turning the plate around in the reconstruction, since for this operation, a slighthly convergent beam would be needed to exactly reverse the light passing through H.

Aberrations coming from L4 have similar consequences: the rays striking H at different angles will reconstruct images with a shift in the distance and unequal magnification. The superimposed images will blur the reconstructed images. This is the case for the figure 8a corresponding to plano-convex lenses L4.

To avoid this defect, the L4 lenses used both for the holographic recording set-up and the reconstruction device are not ordinary lenses like the others, but are spherico-parabolic. The gain in image quality thus obtained by eliminating the spherical aberration is illustrated by the figure 8b.

The figure 8c shows the importance of the value of the hologram aperture on the resti-tuted image resolution. Figure 8c is obtained from the same hologram as figure 8b, but only 15 mm in diameter of H is used, instead of the entire surface for figure 8b. The sharpness of outlines is reduced and the broad areas take on the characteristic speckle appeerence of images formed in laser light.

The figure 9 permits to appreciate the quality of the holographic image of a wristwatch mechanism, 25 mm in diameter, obtained in the same way as the previous example, with the set-up shown in figure 7, i.e. without an objective lens and at a distance of 400 mm from the object.

The film surface used to obtain figure 9 was brought up close to the reconstructed real image by the hologram, until it was in the plane of the mechanical part bearing the engraved inscription. This inscription, with a linear magnification of 10, or a surface area magnification of 100, is given in figure 9a. Figures 9b and c shown two details of the clock movement with the same magnification. For views 9a, b and c, the background irregularities are due not only to the speckle phenomenon, but follow the direction of the part machining and represent the surface roughness of the part. Examining these parts under the microscope, the circular machining striation in photographs 9a and b are about 5 to 10 μm wide. For the gears in figure 9c, the radial striation are very difficult to measure because they are much less than 5 μm in thickness.

In the case of the gliding spark study (previous section) holography serves not only to transport an image, but also to visualize the phenomenon by interferometry. The same is true for the double exposure interferogram of a printed circuit shown in figure 10. The heating of the electronic components of the circuit, while it operates, produces dilatations that the fringes reveal.

Outline objects recording

For this application, the flat mirror M of the previous scheme (figure 7) is suppressed, and the photographic plate holder is disposed in the common part of the two beams E and R (figure 11).

This optical arrangement only allows to record the outline of the studied objects but, in contrary to the case of figure 7, it presents an important advantage: a high coherence is not required for the laser light, because the test beam path lenght is unconnected to the object location. All the small objects included between the collimating lens L4 and the photoplate H (figure 11) can be recorded, whatever the coherence lenght of the laser used may be.

A microscope M, movable along three rectangular axis, makes possible the measurements of the size and space location of the different parts of the 3-D reconstructed image (figure 12).

The reconstructed image can be, of course, also photograhed without objective lens in the same way that described in paragraph 3 (see figure 13a).

The possibilities of recording allowed by the set-up of figure 11 are illustrated by figure 13. For this experiment, horizontal wires, small glass balls and vertical needles, respectively located at 235, 320 and 345 mm of H are simultaneously recorded.

Figure 13a is a general view of the reconstructed real image observed in the plane of horizontal wires; the finest wires (5 μm) are not visible without magnification.

Figures 13b to e show the microscopic examination of the reconstructed images of the three types of objects. The scale of all these views is given by the size of the two wires of figures 13b: 100 and 27 μm in diameter.

The wires of figure 13c have 5 μm in diameter. Figures 13d shows the glass balls (52 μm in diameter) and figure 13e the eye needle.

The high resolution of the reconstructed real image which is possible to obtain is demonstrated by the recording of a microscope stage micrometer (10 microns per subdivision). Figure 14a shows the microscope examination of the holographic image, and figure 14b, for comparison, the direct microscopic examination of the micrometer itself (in same conditions of illumination and magnification).

Flame front study

Figure 15 shows the holographic bench in the combustion laboratory; the studied flame is under the suction-hood[9].

As the optical diagram shows (figure 16), for this experiment the photoplate H is placed in the reference beam only. The test beam passing through the flame does not strike H, but passes beside it. Thus only the light scattered by the powder injected into the flame is received by H and interfers with the reference beam R.

As in the case of the gliding spark (section 2) the light emitted by the object under study (the flame) is negligeable. Because of these photographic conditions, the pictures have a dark background from which the gas jet stands out like a light-coloured smoke, dense when the injected particles are greatest in number and largest in size, but thinned out, in the less seeded areas, or in those areas where the fusion reduces the size of the particles.

Figure 17a shows the jet of gas before ignition. The film used for recording this picture was brought in optical contact with the farthest part of the reconstructed Bunsen burner nozzle.

Figure 17b is also obtained from the same hologram, with the film brought in optical contact with the other side of the Bunsen burner nozzle.

Figure 18 is given by another hologram recorded after ignition of the gas jet: the outline shape is changed. For obtaining this picture, the film was disposed in the same location than for figure 17a.

Figure 19 shows the top of the seeded flame.

By moving the film into the 3-D reconstructed image, we can thus get different cross sections that reveal not only the boundary of the jet for various sections considered, but also internal structure of light and dark areas. This latter result, however, can only be obtained when the particles are far enough apart from each other, and nevertheless numerous enough so that the diffracted light makes the flame visible.

The particle diameter (about 1 μm) is inferior to the recording resolution of the holographic apparatus, thus only few mass of them are visible by microscopic examination.

Conclusion

The holographic device presented in this paper has been first successfully operated for the study of a gliding spark. Without the use of holography, it would have been impossible to measure the diameter of the discharge channel precisely, or to evaluate the refractive index inside it, even approximatively, as it was not feasible to place a microscope lens at few millimeters from the object plane raised to an electric potential of over 100,000 volts.

More generally holography appears as a remote sensing microscopic observation technique. The others various uses of the device presented here, for transparent media and opaque objects recording, demonstrate the versatility of this apparatus, which makes it possible to apply holography as a relay between the phenomenon under study and the instrument of observation and analysis.

In its standard shape, the holographic device can be used to record optical data (light amplitude and phase) in a field 145 mm in diameter, with a resolution equal to that obtained in microscopy for a field at least 20 times smaller (400 times less surface areas) and without the necessity to approach to the phenomenon. But by its design, the apparatus can be modified easily according to the type of phenomenon under study: extent and distance of approach.

The reconstruction device associated to the holographic bench provides, in all cases, a three dimensional image, virtual or real, at the same size than the object. The high resolution real image can be observed, recorded and processed without limitations of observation distance and time duration.

In conclusion, we consider that this holographic equipment is generally suitable for studies requiring remote recording of a maximum of optical data producing a high definition 3-D image easily accessible, whereas the phenomenon itself is not.

References

1. Timko, J.J., The investigation of transport phenomena by applied holography. Proceedings of the Second International Symposium on Flow Visualization, Bochum (RFA), September 9-12, 1980, Hemisphere Publishing Corporation, 1980.
2. Royer, H, La microholographie ultra-rapide et ses applications. Conference at the Colloque de la Société Française de Physique, Clermont-Ferrand, and ISL, report n° CO 204/82, 1982.
3. Smigielski, P., General review on the investigations conducted at ISL in the field of holographic non destructive testing. Lecture given at the Workshop for Industrial Applications of Holographic non Destructive Testing, Brussels, and ISL, report n° CO 203/82, 1982.

4.   Larigaldie, S., Labaune, G. and Moreau, J.P., "Lightning leader laboratory simulation by means of rectilinear surface discharges". J. Appl. Phys., Vol. 52, n° 12, 1981.

5.   Surget, J., Holographic device for rectilinear surface discharge visualization. Third International Symposium on Flow Visualization, Ann Arbor (USA), TP. ONERA n° 1983-104, proceedings by Hemisphere Publishing Corporation, 1983.

6.   Larigaldie, S., Etude expérimentale et modélisation des mécanismes physiques de l'étincelle glissante. Thèse de Doctorat d'Etat, Faculté d'Orsay, n° 3017, june, 1985.

7.   Surget, J., Holographic interferometer for aerodynamic flow analysis. Proceedings of the Second International Symposium on Flow Visualization, Bochum (RFA), september 9-12, 1980, Hemisphere Publishing Corporation, 1980.

8.   Françon, M., Holographie. Masson et Cie, 1980.

9.   Dumont, J.P. and Borghi, R., A study of the structure of turbulent flame. 12th International Symposium on Combustion, University of Michigan, Ann Arbor (USA), 1984.

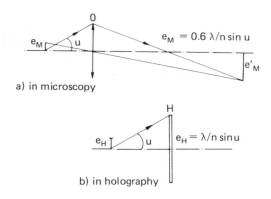

a) in microscopy

$e_M = 0.6\,\lambda/n\sin u$

b) in holography

$e_H = \lambda/n\sin u$

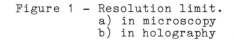

Figure 1 - Resolution limit.
  a) in microscopy
  b) in holography

Figure 2 - Holographic device

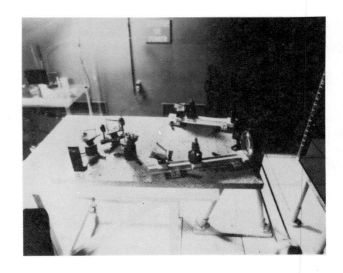

Figure 3 - Holographic device
in the discharge laboratory.

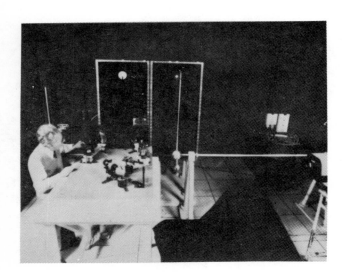

Figure 4 - Optical diagram for
gliding spark study

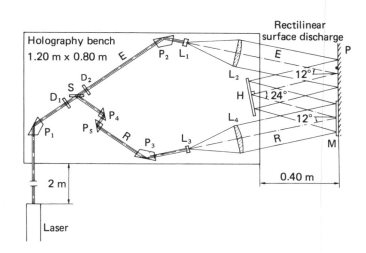

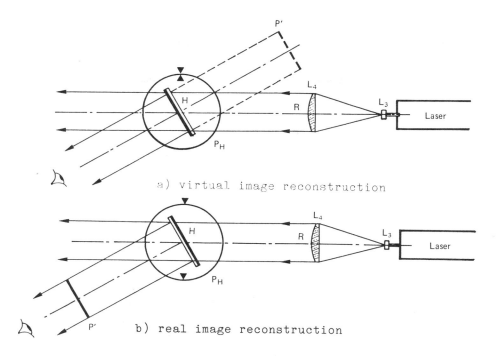

a) virtual image reconstruction

b) real image reconstruction

Figure 5 – Optical diagram of the reconstruction device.

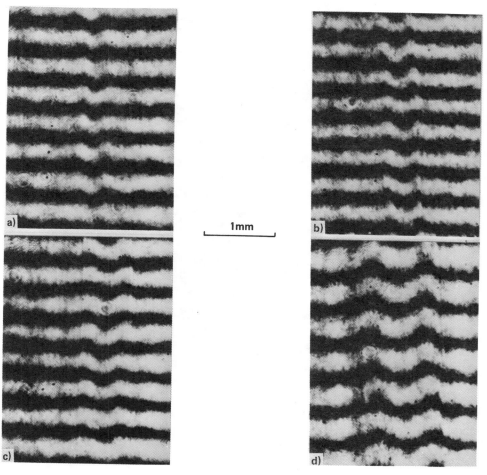

1mm

Figure 6 – Discharge channel finite fringe interferograms
a) ΔT = 115 ns b) ΔT = 145 ns c) ΔT = 200 ns
d) ΔT = 420 ns

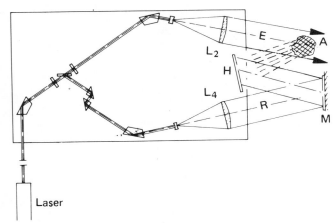

Figure 7 - Optical diagram for opaque objects recording.

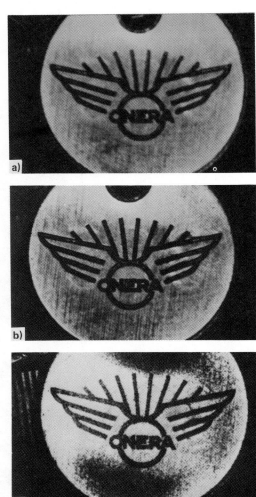

Figure 8 - Effect of the reference beam quality on the reconstructed real images.
a) plano-connex L4 lenses.
b) spherico-parabolic L4 lenses
c) idem b) but with small hologram aperture.

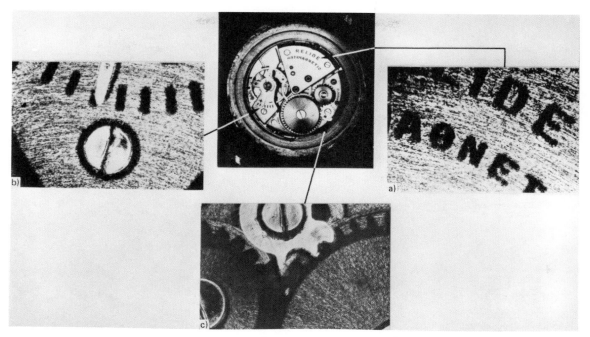

Figure 9 - Wristwatch movement (25 mm in diameter) and magnified details.

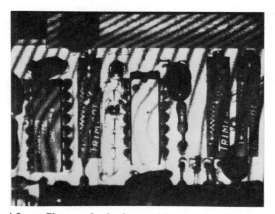

Figure 10 - Thermal deformation of a printed circuit.

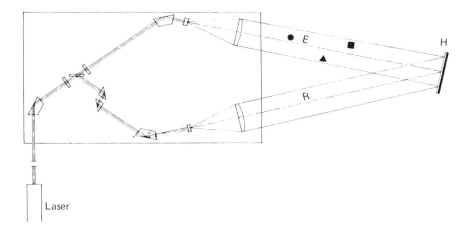

Figure 11 - Optical diagram for outline objects recording.

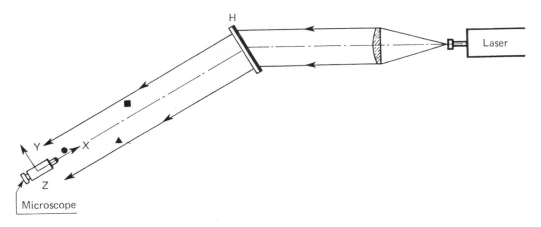

Figure 12 - Reconstructed real image measurement.

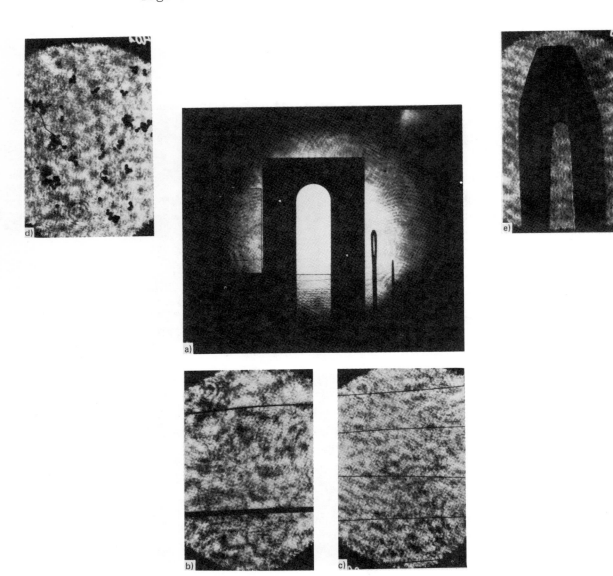

Figure 13 - Reconstructed outline images a) general view b) wires (100 and 27 μm in diameter)
c) wires (5 μm in diameter) d) glass balls (52 μm in diameter) e) eye needle.

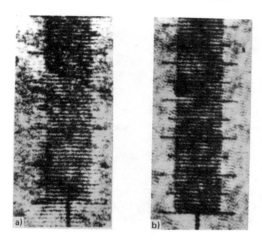

Figure 14 - Microscope stage micrometer
a) holographic image
b) micrometer itself

Figure 15 - Holographic device in
the combustion laboratory

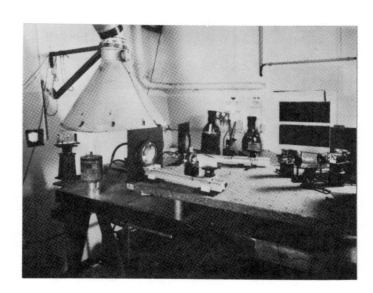

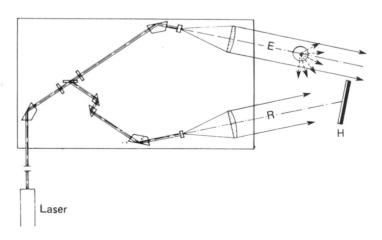

Figure 16 - Optical diagram for front flame study.

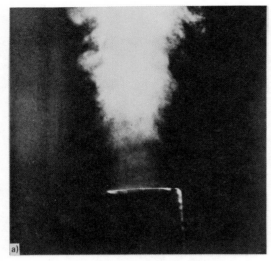 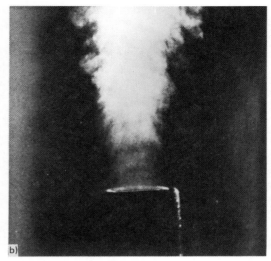

Figure 17 - Feeded gas jet before ignition.
a) First focalization
b) Second focalization

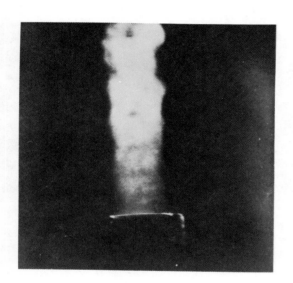

Figure 18 - Same focalization as figure 17a but after ignition.

Figure 19 - Internal examination of a feeded gas jet.

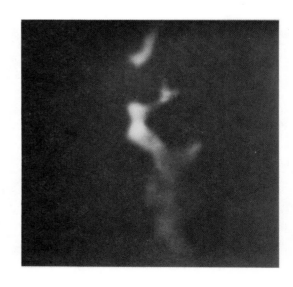

Continuous Wave - Pulse Transfer for High Security Holograms

Simon J.S. Brown

Applied Holographics Plc., Braxted Park, Witham, Essex, CM8 3XB, U.K.

Abstract

The following paper will attempt to highlight the need for security in all walks of life. It will show how holography in general will thwart the conventional counterfeiter, and reflection holography in particular from the Holocopier system will further confound the more determined forger. Mention will be made of the restrictions on copying reflection holograms, and brief mention will be made to the advances to produce such a system. Graphical evidence will be presented to show the degree of control that can and needs to be achieved to ensure high quality, high efficiency copies of original masters by the Holo-copier system.

Introduction

It is now common knowledge that counterfeiting of saleable products accounts for 3 to 6% of world trade - around $60 billion annually. Increasingly the bogus goods are becoming a genuine threat to safety. Now all areas of commerce are looking for ways to ensure that the public receive the services or goods that they are paying for and believe they are receiving. No longer is security restricted to guards in banks or burglar alarm systems. Security means a way of giving confidence that the product purchased is the genuine article. Authentication is another way to term the task.

Any product or facility that can be sold can be counterfeited. It is thus vital that manufacturers have at their disposal obvious ways to distinguish their goods from the usually visually flawless copy. Counterfeiters can produce printed matter so faithfully, even intaglio pringing, water marks etc. can all be simulated to greater or lesser extents by printing.

It is obvious that there is a need for a visually distinctive appendage that is difficult to produce or simulate by conventional printing or photography techniques. Holography offers these unique requirements. Holograms present either striking images or subtle images. They have a mystique that is impossible to simulate, well beyond the scope of conventional forgers and counterfeiters.

Requirements

To be of any use to potential users of this new security feature, the holograms must be available in numbers of up to millions.

The images must also be easily distinguishable. It would be a failure to have similar images on products worth a few pence and many pounds as it may be possible then to purchase the low value goods, extract the hologram and place it on a high value counterfeited product.

We thus require holograms that, if not unique, can be made specially for the various products. The holograms have to be recognised as the authentication device, and this must be able to be affixed to almost any surface or product.

The hologram if it is a security feature, must not be able to sourced from just anywhere, thus these holograms must be obtained from areas concentrating on security printing at least.

Finally, the overriding requirement will be the cost. This added security must not make the product or its packaging prohibitive in terms of cost to the end user. Unit costs must therefore be low for most users.

If all of the above can be met, the general public will expect to see holograms on genuine products and know when forgeries are offered in their place.

This therefore requires and education process of both the general public and the product producers as to what a hologram is and can do.

Existing mass production techniques of holograms

Holography as is well known to this audience stores information in a subtle and cryptic way. The problem is to find a way to produce holograms in commercial numbers. One off's will always be possible using studios and holographic artists. For millions of holograms we need to move to automatic processes away from human restrictions.

If we look at the two main formats for holography to date:

Transmission holography

From the orientation of the interface fringes with respect to the recording medium, this format generally gives rise to a surface modulation in the finished and processed hologram.

This produces a phase grating that can produce highly efficient holograms.

Given that most of the information is encoded in these surface modulations if a hologram can be produced that is a transmission hologram and also white light viewable then the potential to copy it exists.

This is the background to embossed holography, where a rainbow transmission hologram is typically produced that can be considered as having all its holographic information on the surface of the initial recording medium. This is then copied by depositing a metal layer on top of the holographic surface, peeling it away, strengthening it, then using it as a stamp to emboss holographic surface modulations into some flexible metalised surface.

This major technological achievement is now becoming recognised and known to the general public.

The fact that most major credit cards use embossed holograms does not imply that these are the answers to the problem of security as outlined above.

Can they be easily affixed to all products? Can they only be produced by security printers etc? Can they be easily copied?

It is not for me to answer any of the above questions, other than to say, if the information is on the surface of a material, one might assume that it could be copied both physically by contact copying or optically.

Reflection holography. The second major format of holography is reflection holography. Here the information is typically stored in planes parallel to the surface of the recording medium.

Reflection holograms are basically dichroic mirrors, very selective filters. With the information stored inside the bulk of the recording medium, whether it be a photo polymer, ferro electric crystals, photographic emulsion or what ever it can not be violated or copied physically. The only other way to get to the information is optically, the illuminating source will thus have constraints imposed on its coherence and wavelength if a suitable image is to be generated for copying. Already it is becoming obvious that reflection holography ultimately is the answer to the problems outlined above.

Reflection holograms can be made to be both visually attractive as they are almost automatically white light viewable, and yet almost impossible to copy physically or optically. The counterfeiters would have to go to great lengths to copy a transmission hologram, let alone a reflection hologram.

The fact that reflection holograms are so difficult to copy has restricted the retail hologram industry to that of a "cottage" industry. Ways to produce reflection holograms did not, till of late, fit in with requirements of commerce. Costly plant, long individual exposure times, poor quality materials, specialist operation, limited resources, have all kept reflection holography as a "cottage" industry.

Improved security of reflection holograms

Thin film dielectric multi layer stacks and dichroic mirrors are not new, however, these have always been vacuum deposited and uniquely made, hence the high costs and design constraints. It is not difficult to expect that variations in phase many orders of magnitued more complex than simple AR coatings should be difficult to produce in large numbers, let alone copy easily.

The reason lies in the fact that reflection holograms are so selective to both colour and orientation, of the illuminating beam that to copy such a reflected signal it would have to be phase related to some incoming or incident beam. There is thus imposed a coherence restriction in the illuminating source as well.

Imagine then that we have a reflection hologram, that has been tuned to a particular colour. To copy such a hologram, we would need a light source that had a spectral component that was the exact colour the reflection hologram filters out (to within about 10mm) as well as ensuring that the coherence length of this colour was sufficient to result in interference between the reflected signal and incoming beam.

To date I do not know of a source that is both flexible in its spectral composition and still boasts a temporal coherence length of some millimeters.

I include some spectral distribution curves of reflection holograms specially tuned by us to allow us to copy them at the common wavelengths of 694, 633 and the same image tuned down to 550nm. It can be seen that the spectral distributions have maintained a fairly narrow bandwidth (30mm) and the efficiency of subsequent copies depends strongly on the peak of the distribution lying with $\pm$ 10nm of the desired location.

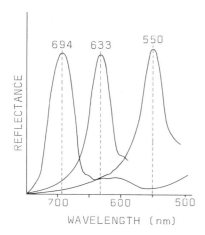

GRAPH 1

Spectral distribution showing master tuning

We have developed techniques for the accurate tuning of reflection holograms to allow highly efficient copying. This is obviously a major achievement and closely guarded by Applied Holographics. This does not however indicate how it is possible to mass replicate these holograms, and yet maintain the viewability and security of the image.

Mass production of reflection holograms by the Holocopier

To mass produce reflection holograms requires a complete rethink of the ways such holograms have typically been made.

Mass production has to be done optically since the information can not be extracted physically. The light source must be powerful enough to "expose" the recording medium quickly and efficiently. The recording will probably be done one at a time to maintain quality; in direct contrast with conventional techniques. The following was therefore proposed

1) Change the recording light source: CW lasers are good for origination, however, they are slow. A pulse laser is powerful, it can expose a suitably sensitised medium in a fraction of a second removing constraints on stability

Exposure areas can thus be in areas of vibration, and individual exposures need only be seconds apart (if that). Temporal coherence is also no problem with a pulses laser.

2) Change the recording medium. To date the 'fastest' recording media have been photographic silver halide based emulsions. Quality control has however been questioned as batch to batch reliability is in general poor in existing products.

The presentation format has also not been in keeping with mass production. What is needed is a silver halide based emulsion that is presented on rolls, that has been produced with good quality control to ensure high batch to batch repeatability, plus reliability, as well as good control of the grain size to minimize scatter and noise. It is also desirable to have this emulsion sensitised specifically for the pulse laser chosen to perform the mass productions.

3) Processing. If a silver halide emulsion is chosen it will have to be wet processed to maintainquality and the idea of mass production, this will have to be done automatically.

This brings the problem of developing a chemistry that is both suitable for an automatic processing system, with its associated environmental constraints, and also produces highly efficient holograms at the end.

4) Finishing. The resultant holograms will need to be finished by lamination, die-cutting and label making techniques if the above mentioned constraints of the security device are to be met.

The above series of problems and suggested solutions have been brought together as the Applied Holographics Holocopier.

This system includes a specially modified pulsed ruby laser, housed inside a specially designed exposure chamber. Here the specially produced Applied Holographics Holofilm, which is now recognised as being the best holographic emulsion available in terms of resolution and diffraction efficiency, is used to record either reflection holograms directly from models, or copy either transmission masters or specially produced reflection masters.

Production rates so far of 350,000 cm^2 per hour can be achieved per system.

From here the exposed Holofilm is passed to the automatic processor, which is again a specially manufactured piece of hardware to meet the needs of holographic emulsions. The chemistry is unique to Applied Holographics and is produced under the trade name Holochem. This chemistry is produced in concentrate form that has again high quality control in its production to ensure high batch to batch repeatability, a long shelf life and long life inside the automatic processor. (In production the chemistry is changed at 3 month intervals).

The processed rolls of Holofilm are then laminated, die-cut and finished to produce thousands of holographic sticky labels that can be treated as any other label and fixed to almost any product, package or security document.

Again this lamination device has had to be specially produced to meet the exacting needs of holography and security. Included in this device is a registration mechanism to locate the holographic image to a high degree of accuracy repeatably.

Thus a Holocopier mass production system consists of an exposure chamber, housing a pulsed ruby laser, a processing system, a finishing system. It uses uniquely produced consumables of film and chemistry and lamination materials (backings and adhesives). All of the above are suitably covered by patents and confidentiality agreements.

C.W. Pulse transfer techniques

The Holocopier system can originate reflection holograms from models. These can be processed to give final holograms that lie well away from existing laser lines that could be used to attempt to copy them.

The figures overleaf show how the same hologram can be processed to appear red, gold or green.

Note how the images have been machine tuned to the He-Ne wavelength, and equally as easily away from the common lines of argon and He-Ne. Now even we could not copy these.

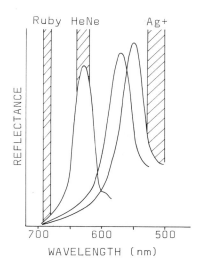

GRAPH 2

Spectral distributions showing automatic
processor tuning

The problem is then, well if the hologram cannot be copied, can not the model be remade and a few similar copies made by conventional means?

Would this then question the security aspects of reflection holograpy?

The Holocopier however, does allow the copying of reflection masters. These can be made carefully by holographic artists to be visually distinctive yet very difficult to see how to reproduce.

This therefore necessitates the production of the H1 and/or H2 using a standard CW laser source. this is then processed to tune the peak response of the hologram to 694nm. Using CW lasers allows the originator to create exactly the illusion he wishes. The processing and subsequent copying maintains faithfully the stored information as the shown spectral curves demonstrate.

For security purposes it is thus possible to incorporate in the finished hologram both CW master hologram information and information from a model that can be incremented between exposures. This allows the possibility of making each hologram unique, enhancing its security potential.

It is also possible to make the final hologram in at least two discrete colours, causing the potential counterfeiter more headaches. This is done automatically in the exposure of the hologram and involves no pre-swelling of the layer. Colour tuning obviously depends on the optical path difference between the reflecting planes, allowing this to be altered by physically changing the spacing or by modifying the refractive index modulation across the hologram. Typically this effect is achieved by accident, however, our control of this feature offers tremendous possibilities for the security use of reflection holography.

It is tempting to say that such holograms are impossible to copy, we will however be more realistic and say that reflection holograms produced by the Holocopier for security purposes will be very difficult to copy and will ensure some marked increase in the potential security of any product, package or document.

Such holographic labels can also embellish and enhance products, giving security as well as a most attractive effect. Do not ignore the tremendous public interest in holographic images in general.

Conclusion

We have shown how security is beginning to affect us all in everyday circumstances.

Counterfeiting risks our very safety. Producers need to have access to ways to authenticate the genuine article that are very difficult to simulate.

Reflection holography in particular offers such possibilities. The Applied Holographics Holocopier system can produce such holograms in commercial numbers and at realistic rates.

High security labels can be purchased for a few pence to protect almost any product or package. Low cost, high security is now available.

In-line far-field holography and diffraction pattern analysis : new developments

Özkul C., Allano D., Trinité M., Anthore N.

Université de Rouen - U.A. CNRS 230 - Faculté des Sciences
C.O.R.I.A.
B.P. 67   76130 Mont-Saint-Aignan   (France)

Abstract

A holographic recording with a filter is studied. In particular, influences of the hologram finite aperture on filtered images are considered. Irradiance distribution in defocused image is calculated. Furthermore in application an instrument measuring the diameter and 3-D position of a glass fiber is described.

Introduction

In the first part of this communication, we are dealing with the filtering during in-line holographic recording and with the calculation of irradiance distribution in the reconstruted images. The aim of the filtering during the recording is increasing the contrast of the high frequency fringes of far-field diffraction patterns, thus increasing the field depth. The subject matter has been adressed in the recent publications [1,2,3,4].

After a brief review, the influence of the hologram transfer function on the reconstructed image will constitute a focus point in this paper [5].

In the second part, we will be interested in the description of an instrument which measures the diameter of a glass-fiber being drawn out. The functioning principle of this instrument is based on the computation of irradiance distributions with the far-field diffraction formalism wich is used for a long time to describe the intensity recorded on the hologram. Basically, the instrument contains a photodiodes array as receiver instead of the holographic plate. It allows to extract directly the informations carried by the diffracted field for measuring the diameter and space coordinates of the object whereas the hologram transforms the diffracted field to an image for giving the same informations.

Part 1 : Filtering during the hologram recording

The sample volume is imaged near the hologram plate. Here, one-dimensional opaque objects are considered : they are illuminated with a spherical wave Σ which converges on the filter coating at the center of the objective. For simplification, the image magnification is assumed to be unity. The diameter of the object is 2a. Figures 1 (a) and (b) show the coordinate systems.

Neglecting the phase term due to the filter, the amplitude transmittance of the diffracting aperture is

$$b(x_1) = \text{rect}\,(x_1/2b) + (\alpha-1).\text{rect}\,(x_1/2b\beta)$$

where 2b and 2bβ are the geometrical apertures of the lens and filter coating.

The hologram is formed by recording the interferences between the field diffracted by the object and the background attenuated by the filter.

The wavelength λ and the radius Z_s of the wave front curvature are taken as having the same values during hologram recording and reconstruction phases.

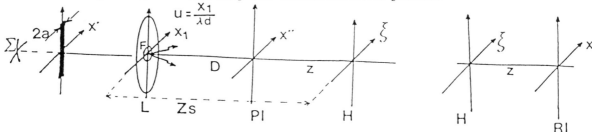

Figure 1

(a) Recording geometry : PI projected image plane, H hologram plate, L relay lens, F filter coating

(b) Reconstruction geometry : H Hologram, RI reconstructed image plane

Irradiance distribution at recording plane

The exact calculation of the irradiance distribution at recording plane is described elsewhere [1,2]. Main results are put in evidence by two examples :

The first example concerns an opaque wire of 60μm in diameter, lying at a distance 2f from the relay lens (f : 105mm, N = 4.5). The diameter of the filter coating is equal to 0.3 b and its intensity transmittance α^2 is equal to 0.04. The filtered image is formed at a distance Z = 200mm from the hologram plate. The irradiance distribution following ξ-axis is plotted on Figure 2. The central lobe of the diffraction pattern from the abscissa $\xi = -1530\mu m$ up to $\xi = 1530\mu m$ can be described by classical formula[6].

$$I_1(\xi) = \alpha^2 \{1 - C_1 \, F_1(\xi) + C_2 \, F_2^{\,2}(\xi)\} \qquad (1)$$

where

$$C_1 = \frac{4a}{\sqrt{\lambda ZR}} \qquad C_2 = \frac{4a^2}{\lambda ZR} \qquad R = \frac{Z_s}{Z_s - Z}$$

$$F_1(\xi) = \cos\left(\frac{\pi \xi^2}{\lambda ZR} - \frac{\pi}{4}\right) \cdot F_2(\xi) \qquad F_2(\xi) = \frac{\sin\left(\frac{2\pi a\xi}{\lambda Z}\right)}{\left(\frac{2\pi a\xi}{\lambda Z}\right)}$$

The intensity distribution corresponding to encircled region and in its symmetry can be approximated by sinusoidal portions chosen with adequate amplitudes. Outside preceding intervals, the following equation is considered

$$I_2(\xi) = \alpha^2 - \alpha C_1 \cdot F_1(\xi) + C_2 \cdot F_2^{\,2}(\xi) \qquad (2)$$

Our second example is an opaque wire of 50μm in diameter. The other parameters are : f = 150mm, N = 3, β = 0.008, α^2 = 0.25, Z = 200mm.

The irradiance distribution in diffraction pattern corresponding to this example is plotted in Figure 3. It can be approximated by :

$$I_3(\xi) = I_2(\xi) \cdot \left(1 + \varepsilon \, \frac{\sin\left(3.2 \, \frac{2\pi a\xi}{\lambda Z}\right)}{\left(3.2 \, \frac{2\pi a\xi}{\lambda Z}\right)}\right) \qquad (3)$$

where $I_2(\xi)$ is as defined in equation (2). ε is taken equal to 0.19 in the interval |400μm, 500μm| and equal to 0.35 outside of this interval.

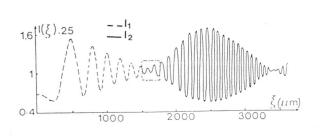

Figure 2

Intensity distribution in diffraction pattern to be recorded 2a = 60μm, Z = 200mm, Z_s = 410mm, β = 0.15 α = 0.2

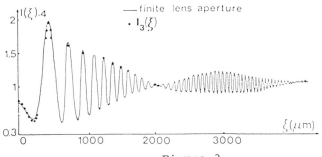

Figure 3

Irradiance distribution in diffraction pattern   2a = 50μm, α = 0.5, β = 0.008, Z = 200mm Z_s = 500mm

Irradiance distribution in reconstructed images : effect of the finite hologram aperture

The calculation of the reconstructed images without taking into account the finite aperture of the hologram is published elsewhere[2]. Here, we assume that the hologram can be considered as a finite aperture for low contrast-high frequency fringes of the diffraction pattern.

The amplitude transmittance of the hologram is given by the equation :

$$t(\xi) = t_B - K \, H(\xi) \cdot I(\xi) \qquad (4)$$

Here K is a constant and t_b is the intercept of the linear portion of the t-E curve with the t axis. $H(\xi)$ represents an infinite aperture for the constant part of the intensity $I(\xi)$, but a finite aperture for the variable part of $I(\xi)$. Considering the latter case $H(\xi)$ will be defined as :

$$H(\xi) = 1 \quad \text{in the interval} \quad \left| - n \frac{\lambda Z}{2a} \ , \ n \frac{\lambda Z}{2a} \right|, \ H(\xi) = 0 \text{ out of this interval}$$

Taking $n = 1,2,3$ we are getting the image evolution when the aperture dimension increases from the central lobe of the diffraction pattern to the outside lobes.

Amplitude distribution following x-axis of the reconstructed image plane at a distance Z from the hologram (see Figure 1-b), is given by :

$$A(x) = \int_{-\infty}^{\infty} \left| t_B - K.H(\xi) \ I(\xi) \right| \ \exp \left| \frac{i\pi}{\lambda Z} (x-\xi)^2 - \frac{i\pi}{\lambda Z_S} \xi^2 \right| \ d\xi \qquad (5)$$

The integral A(x) is computed using the analytical functions defined in previous section for replacing $I(\xi)$. The intensity distribution in reconstructed image is also expressed as

$$I(x) = A(x) \ A^*(x) \qquad\qquad (6)$$

Theoretical curves of the Figures 4 correspond to our first example ($2a = 60\mu m$, $\alpha^2 = 0.04$, $Z = 200mm$). The serie (4a) is obtained with $p = t_B/K - 1 = 0.1$ and the serie (4b) with $p = 0.3$. It is to point out that p indicates the average exposure level of the hologram.

Figures 5 correspond to our second example ($2a = 50\mu m$, $\alpha^2 = 0.25$, $Z = 200mm$).

Examination of these curves leads to four remarks :

i)   image contrast is better with $p = 0.1$ than with $p = 0.3$ consequently, the hologram must be overexposed

ii) the image edge sharpness increases with n, that is to say, with increasing the hologram aperture (use of filter is made for this aim)

iii) in the case of the first example (small value of α, large value of β), the image is very different from those obtained without filtering. In particular, the maximum intensity in image increase with n.

iiii) In the case of the second example (large value of α, small value of β), the image form is similar to those obtained without filtering.

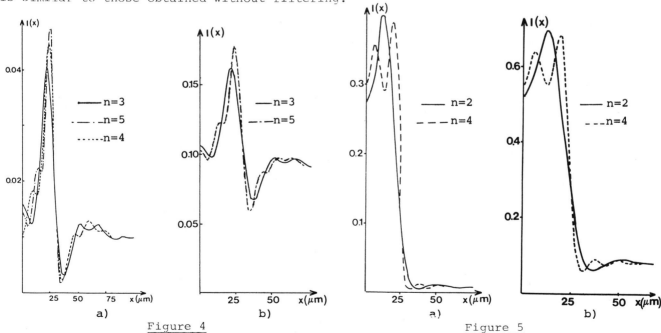

Figure 4   Figure 5

Irradiance distribution in reconstructed images with finite hologram aperture

4) $2a=60\mu m$, $\alpha=0.2$ $\beta=0.15$ 5) $2a=50\mu m$ $\alpha=0.5$ $\beta=0.008$

a- $p=0.1$ b- $p=0.3$ a- $p=0.1$ b- $p=0.3$

Irradiance distribution in defocused reconstructed images

The reconstructed image is defocused when a plane located at a distance Z_O (not equal to Z) from the hologram plane is considered. The amplitude distribution in this plane can be computed replacing Z in exponent term of the equation (5) by Z_O.

The intensity in defocused image is then given with help of the equation (6).

Figures 6 show the image evolution with $\Delta Z = Z_O-Z$ in the first example, respectively for p = 0.1 and p = 0.3. The maximum value of the intensity and the sharpness of the image edge decrease when ΔZ increases. This suggests in particular that, the focusing plane can be found by searching the maximum value of the intensity with an automatic system. For such systems, the evaluation of the maximum slope is not easy compared to the determination of the maximum intensity.

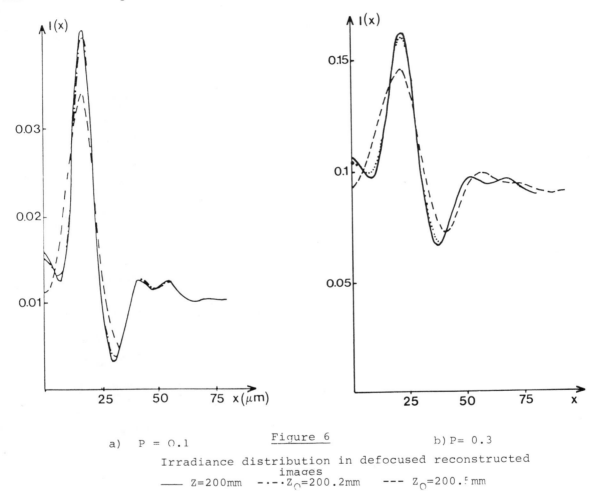

a)   P = 0.1   Figure 6   b) P= 0.3

Irradiance distribution in defocused reconstructed
images
—— Z=200mm   -·-·Z_O=200.2mm   --- Z_O=200.5mm

Experimental result

Experiments are performed for holographic recording of a wire of 10µm in diameter, 200mm away from the hologram plate with filter coating having a relative aperture β equal to 0.15 and a real amplitude transmittance α equal to 0.2. It is worth to notice that Z > 1000 d^2/λ. This value is to be compared with those obtained without filtering (Z < 200 d^2/λ).

Part. II : Automatic measurement process of both the diameter and the 3D position of glass fibers

An optical setting (see Figure 7) similar to that of the Figure 1 where the photosensitive film is replaced by a photodiode array (Thomson TH 7831 CD, 1728 diodes) has been used without filter.

The diffraction pattern of the object is directly sampled with this detector with a sampling step of 13μm.

When the central lobe of the diffraction pattern is explored, an experimental sampling resolution equal to the image diameter (2.a.γ) is required.

The magnification of the setting is scaled by drawing the curve γ = f(Z) for test-objects. (Z is the distance between the image and the receiver).

For the moving objects as for the fiber being drawn out, the distance Z is first computed using the abscissa where the intensity is equal to unity. After that, the magnification and then the position in the object space are deduced with the help of that scaling curve.

In order to use the far-field diffraction formalism, the measurement domain is limited to the range of diameters for which the inequation FRAU = $(2a\gamma)^2/(\lambda Z) < 0.2$ holds.

For reconciling the Fraunhofer condition, the required sampling resolution, and the fiber movement amplitude, two measuring ranges have been chosen : i):5-10μm ii):10-25μm

The minimal magnification of the setting is fixed for the inferior limit of each range, taking into account the sampling step, (2aγ > 5 steps). The superior limit of the diameter ranges is then determined by the maximal displacement of the object, knowing that the new values of Z and γ resulted from this displacement should not violate the Fraunhofer's condition.

For example, in first measuring range (i) the minimal magnification is fixed at γ = 12 considering the minimal diameter of 5μm, also a maximal diameter of 10μm results assuming a longitudinal shift equal to 0.5mm following optical axis in object space.

The Figure 8 shows the minimum and maximum values of Z in each measuring range as a function of the diameter for a given value of the parameter γ_m.

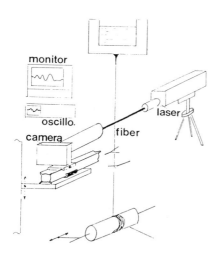

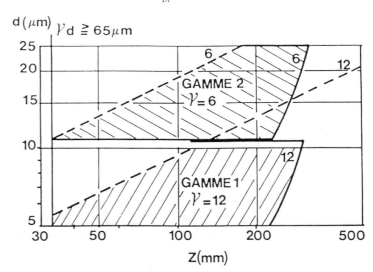

Figure 7

Optical arrangement on the industrial site

Figure 8 : Z_{max} and Z_{min} as a function of d

- in dashed line, minimal value of Z corresponding to Frau = 0.2 ($Z_{mini} = 5 \cdot (\gamma d)^2/\lambda$) for γ=6 and γ=12

- in continuous line, superior limit of Z, for an analysis of the central diffraction lobe assuming a displacement in depth of 0.5mm for the fiber

Principle of the measurement

The photometric signal to be processed results of three successive recordings.
i)   Obscurity signal (black : N_J)
ii) Signal received by the detector in the absence of the object (white A_J)
iii) Signal received by the detector in the presence of the object (B_J)

From N_J, A_J, B_J, a function $Y_J = \dfrac{B_J - N_J}{A_J - N_J}$ is deduced for each photodiode (J)

In our experiments, $0 < Y_J < 2$ and the incremental step of measure has been equal to 0.01
The synoptic in Figure 9 outlines the measurement set. After reception, the digital photometric signal is displayed. This interactive system allows the experimentor to decide,
or not, about the storage on disc and the following processing.

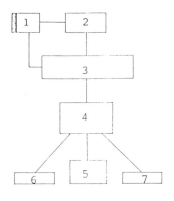

D - detector TH 7831 CD. THOMSON

1 - analog video kit. THOMSON

2 - amplifier (tunable threshold) CORIA

3 - digital oscilloscope. NICOLET

4 - micro-computer 64K. APPLE II e

5 - display monitor

6 - floppy disque

7 - image writer printer

Figure 9

Data acquisition and processing

Processing of the photometric data

It consists of the determination of the minimum, maximum and zero of the function
$(1 - Y_J)$ and the attempt to obtain the best adequation to the model of Fraunhofer. As an
example, the Figure 10 shows sample signals compared to the value calculated for a calibrated wire.

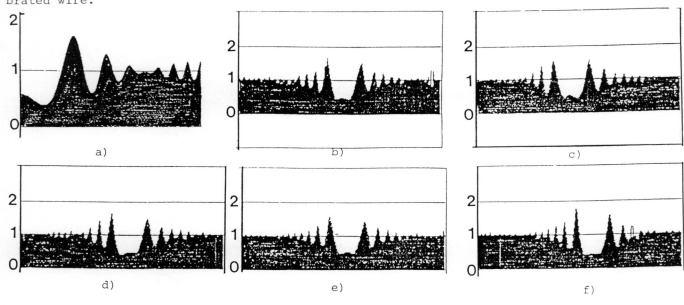

Figure 10

a) Theoretical curve : $2a = 8,7\mu m$, $Z = 96,5mm$ $\lambda = 0.63\mu m$ $Z_S = 607mm$ FRAU = 0.12

b - f) Sampled photometric signals after processing

The synoptic in Figure 11 shows different stages of processing :
i)   computing the distance Z
ii) computing the exact value of the transversal magnification (for a given range of diameters)
iii) computing the diameter d.

During the experimentations in the laboratory, the instrument under design (with continuous laser He-Ne of 5mW) made it possible to measure with a 10% precision in a single scan (in a reproducible way) for the diameter range of 5-25µm. It has also been tested in the factory on glass-fibers in movement.

To improve the precision of measures, it is necessary to reduce the exposure length of photodiodes and to cumulate the sucessive scannings of the detector. In other hand in order to increase signal noise ratio, the filtering method described in first part of this paper   can be used.

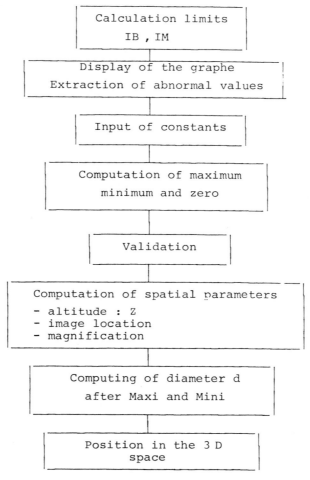

Figure 11

Flowchart for the processing of photometric data to compute
the diameter and the position
of the fiber

Conclusion

Use of a semi-transparent filter during in-line far-field holographic recording makes the hologram aperture more large. Thus, the image contrast and the sharpness of the image edge increase. As an application of calculation of the irradiance recorded on holographic plate, an instrument measuring the diameter of a glass in fiberisation process is described. This instrument is to be improved by new progress in scaning method and in both optical and numerical signal processings.

References

1. Ozkul C., "Imagerie par un objectif avec une obstruction centrale semi-transparente et application à la microholographie", J. of Optics (Paris), vol. 16, N° 1, pp. 29-35, 1985.
2. Ozkul C., Allano D., "Amélioration de la profondeur de champ en microholographie pour un objet de diamètre donné, Actes du Colloque National de Visualisation et de Traitement d'images, 15-17 Janvier 1985 - Nancy - France.
3. Ozkul C., Allano D., Trinité M., "Filtering effects in far-field in-line holography and in diffraction pattern analysis", Proceedings of SPIE's, 29th annual International Technical Symposium, 18-23 August 1985, San-Diego.
4. Molesini G., Bertrani D., Cetica M., "In line holography with interference filters as Fourier processors", Optica Acta, Vol. 29, n° 4, pp. 479-484, 1982.
5. Ozkul C., "Effects of the finite aperture on the linewidth measurement using in-line Fraunhofer holography, Optics and Laser Techno. To be published.
6. Tyler G.A., Thompson N.J., "Fraunhofer holography applied to particle size analysis. A reassessment", Optica Acta, Vol. 23, n° 9, pp. 685-700, 1976.

3-D Holographic Miniprojector Used for Micro-
circuits Assembly and Quality Control

Xu Kun-xian

Shanghai Institute of Laser Technology
319 Yue Yang Road, Shanghai 200031
People's Republic of China

Abstract

A 3-D holographic miniprojector on the basis of holographic(optical element) screens using
for integrated circuits assembly and quality control is described. This is a compact, profe-
ssional projection-type microscope using hybrid technique combing the advantages of both stereoscopy and holography. The optical principle and system of this miniprojector, recording
scheme of holographic diffusing screen, improvement of chromatic dispersion of screen and characteristics of projection system are discussed.

Introduction

Up to the present, the visual inspection and assembly operation of minicomponents such as
integrated circuits, printed boards and precise metals etc. in the industrial departments still use general binocular stereomicroscope(BSM). However, the microscope observation would
result in considerable visual and overall fatigue of the microscope operators. This in turn
has a deleterious effect on labour productivity and product quality.

One method of reducing the visual and general fatigue when working with a microscope is to
project the image of the object onto a translucent screen, which provides more comfortable
viewing conditions compared with looking through the exit pupils of the eyepices of a microscope. However, the transmission-type diffusing screens used in the visual-optical instruments
uniformly diffuse light flux at a wide angle so that only a small portion of it enters the
spectator pupils. The rest of the light being wasted. The brilliance of screen images are very
dark. Meanwhile, this diffusing screen can also not form stereoscopic observation of 3-D screen images.

The stereoscopic techniques on the basis of simultaneous vision of 2-D images leading to a
3-D perception of the scene and the holographic techniques on the basis of the coding of the
object information in form of interference fringes are certainly the efficient techniques(1)
for providing a 3-D visualization of objects. Unfortunately, both of the stereoscopy and holography must be used more complex coding and decoding process of object information. The holographic step is sensitive to external perturbations and most always be achieved in strict
stability conditions. Moreover, for retrieving the object information it is necessary to de-
code the information recorded in the hologram using the expensive laser. The stereoscopic
techniques needs perfect independence between the two reflected beams containing the information of each images so that it must use a particular coding of the two projected images such
as chromatic or polarization coding. The decoding being performed with suitable spectacles
such as chromatic filters or polarizers(2). Therefore, it is important to develop a another
more promising stereoscopic technique.

The Optical Principle and configuration of 3-D Holographic Miniprojector

In this paper we propose a hybrid technique combing the advantages of both stereoscopy and
holography. The principle is based on the projecting two 2-D images magnified from BSM objectives and projection oculars on the holographic diffusing screen(HDS) recorded by lensless
Fourier transform hologram(Fig.1). Thanks to the well-known focusing and strict directional
diffusing properties of holographic optical element(HOE) it is possible to make up stereo effect of separation of both channels so that two viewing zones are formed for the left and right eyes separately. In other words, HDS scatter the incident light in precise directions and

can even posses various independent diffusion function, each of them transmitting certain information. It is obvious that a screen with such properties may avoid the coding and decoding process of conventional stereoscopic techniques.

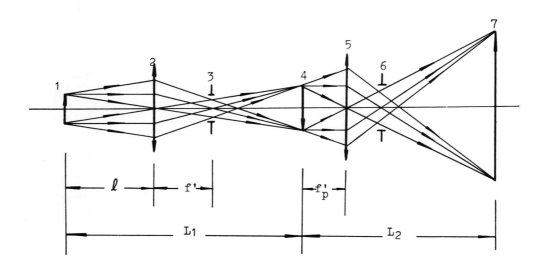

Fig.1. The optical principle of 3-D holographic miniprojector
1. object, 2. BSM objective, 3,6 diaphragm 4. intermediate image, 5. projection lens, 7. HDS.

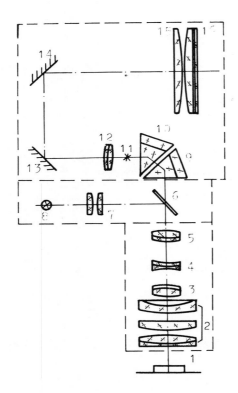

1. minicomponents,
2. 1 X objective,
3. change magnification objective
4. compensation objective,
5. stationary objective,
6. semi-transparent plate,
7. condenser lens,
8. halogen bulb(12V/50W),
9,10. Schmidt prisms,
11.intermediate image,
12.projection ocular,
13,14. mirrors,
15. collector lens,
16. HDS.

Fig.2. The configuration of 3-D HMP

The configuration of 3-D HMP is schematized in Fig.2. The minicomponents to be inspected is illuminated by coaxial incident light from built-in illuminator consisted of a point source 8, condenser lens 7 and semitransparent plate 6. The illuminated minicomponent is doubly magnified by BSM objective A and projection ocular 12 up to HDS 16 sizes. The HDS transforms the projected image to a screen image, which the viewer can observe viewing zone of HDS. In order to raising the brilliance of screen images, and taking pupils transformation, the collector lenses 15 closely spaced with HDS is placed. The combined action of the collector lenses and the HDS result in the fact that the exit pupils of projection system, which has a diameter of about 1 mm, are transformed into two monocular viewing zone having a diameter of 60 mm, located at a distance of 250 mm(i.e. normal visual distance) from the screen. The distance between the center of the zones is equal to 60 mm, it approximately matches the average eye base. Therefore, the operating conditions of a HMP are that of a stereomicroscope with a viewing zone and with the additional possibility of continuous seeing in the round the 3-D image within the viewing zones. Moreover, the large dimensions of the zones(compared with the exit pupils of the microscope) give the operator some freedom of movement with respect to the screen. This contributes to a relaxation of the operator's posture and reduces fatigue.

This apparatus is illuminated by coaxial incident illuminator with 12V/50W halogen blub. The coaxial illuminator enables flat specular objects, which frequently occur in electronics and metallurgy, to be observed. Due to the light from a 12V/50W halogen bulb is directed along the two beam paths in the stereomicroscope so that the structure of semiconductor components and of metal sections are seen, sometimes as interference colours. It is possible to increasing visual sensitivity and resolution power of eyes.

Recording Scheme of Holographic Diffusing Screen

The holographic screens(3) consisted of HOE can focus the images projected on it into given viewing zones. It has higher brilliance of screen images compared to general diffusing screen, However, because of undiffraction radiation (zero order beam) for transmission-type holographic screen, it is possible to observe exit pupils of projection objectives. In order to overcome above disadvantage, it is necessary to use HDS with focusing characteristics. The operation principle of HDS may be considered as combination effect of both a focusing hologram and a diffuser(such as ground glass)(4).

The HDS may be recorded by recording geometry of lensless Fourier transform hologram. The recording geometry of HDS of lensless Fourier transform hologram is schematized in Fig.3. The

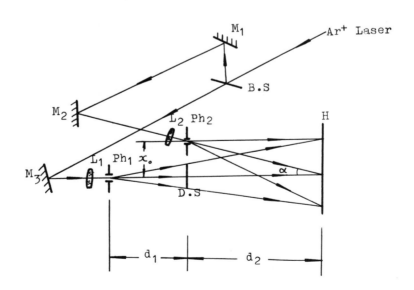

Figure.3. The HDS'recording geometry of lensless Fourier
transform hologram
B.S. beam splitter, M₁, M₂, M₃ mirrors,
L₁,L₂ microscope objectives, Ph₁,Ph₂
pinhole filters,D.S. diffusing screen,
H DCG plate.

wavelength 514.5 nm from an argon-ion laser is splitted by beam splitter B.S. into object and reference beam. The object beam is reflected by mirror M_3. Then, expanded beam passed through point source consisting of microscope objective L_1 and pin hole filter Ph_1 is projected on the ground glass diffuser. The diffusing light scattered by diffuser is further projected on the dichromatic gelation (DCG) plate H. The reference beam is reflected by mirrors M_1 and M_2. Then. expanded beam passed through point source consisting of microscope objective L_2 and pin hole filter Ph_2 placed in the diffuser plane is directly projected on the DCG plate. After developing, the resulting hologram is a lensless Fourier transform hologram. The HDS studied in this paper use Fourier transform hologram screens. Its recording parameters are as follows (refer to Fig.3.). The distance from pinhole filter to diffuser $d_1=178$ mm, the distance from diffuse to DCG plate $d_2=250$ mm, the distance from reference source to center of diffuser $X_0 =60$ mm, the angle between object and reference beam $\alpha =13°30'$.

The hardened DCG plates used hardening agent of 0.5% ammonium dichromate and sensitized by means of 3-5% aqueous solution of $(NH_4)_2Cr_2O_7$ is prepared by gravitation method for appling the gelatin to the glass. After the exposure of DCG plate, the plate is pretreat by KodaKF9 rapid fixer firstly. Then, it is developed in heat running water($47°C$). The third step is immersed it in different proportional mixture of isopropyl alcohol and water, so as to dries the layer extremely rapidly. The final step is fixed by dry in the heat-wind. This hologram screen processed by above steps has high diffraction efficiency and low noise. In addition, in order to protect the DCG emulsion layer from mechanical damage and the influence of the ambient humidity a cover glass was cemented on the emulsion side of the hologram.

In order to realize reconstruction of Fourier transform hologram. We must produce Fourier transform of hologram. This can be realized by using Fraunhofer diffraction pattern of hologram. Fourier transform may be also viewed in the focus plane of lens illuminated by collimated beams[5]. As shown in Fig.4, if hologram is directly placed behind the lens with focus length f'. the zero order beam is positioned in the focus of focus plane. The two sides of

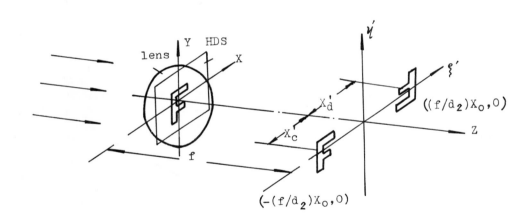

Fig.4. The reconstruction of real image of lensless Fourier transform hologram

optical axis are two reconstructed images. The real image and its conjugate image are symmetry on optical axis. The real image is reverse and its center position is locate at $X'd=(f'/d_2) X_0$. The conjugate image is right and its center position is locate at $X'_C = -(f/d_2)X_0$.

Now, let us consider the operating principle of HDS in the HMP(refer to Fig.5). When the screen is illuminated by reconstructed beam from exit pupils of projection ocular. The HDS diffract incident beam into zero order (undiffraction beam) beam and ±1 order diffraction beam. The geometry of hologram is so arrangemented that the direction of reconstructed + 1 order beam is proceeded along direction of optical axis. Meanwhile, the zero order beam and -1 order diffraction beam are parasitic and are removed by means of optic tube and diaphragm. In addition, the collector lens contacted with HDS is positioned in front of the HDS. There are two purposes. One is that it can be transformed exit pupil of projection ocular into the viewing zone(i.e. the exit pupil image of projection ocular). The another is that the second lens of condenser system received the parallel beams is served as reconstruction lens of Fourier transform hologram. Therefore, the viewing zones and diffuser images reconstructed from the HDS are placed in the focus plane of reconstruction lens.

As far as the common sense is concerned, the operating conditions of HMP are that of a stereomicroscope with an eyepiece pupil and with the additional possibility of continuous seeing in the round the 3-D image within the viewing zone. Such a projection-type holographic

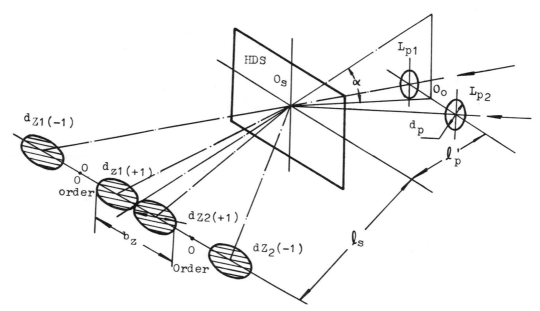

Fig.5. The operating principle for 3-D HMP

microscope have high screen image illuminance and clear separation of perspectives in the viewing zone.

However, because of hypertrophic image distortion caused by square magnification of the longitudinal coordinate, only a small increase(about 10 times) is admissible for known holographic projection system, with greater magnification a problem arises. Since the aperture diameter of the projection optics get smaller, the size of the viewing zone, representing the image of that aperture on the screen, becomes too narrow for binocular seeing round the screen image. Therefore, it can not satisfy observing condition of binocular vision.

When analysing the structure of the viewing zone for binocular vision, it is easy to know that its horizontal demensions have to be bigger than the vertical one.This points to fact that one big projection aperture may be replaced by a horizontal row of two(or more than two) aperture of smaller diameter, altogether ensuring the require width b_z of the viewing zone. Therefore, the holographic miniprojector proposed in this paper is practically a projector of which the viewing zones are formed for the left and right eyes separately..In other words, it is a double-lens projection system. Such a projection system permit $dZ \leq$ beye, here, dZ is the width of the subzone, beye is the mean value of the eye pupil diameters. It may even be $dZ \ll$ beye that is to say, break between the left and right zones is admissible. This relaxes the rigidity of the requirements on the parameters of all lenses since it becomes possible to change the parameters of a separate subzone which may vary from beye to zero(as in the case of stereoscope or binoculars).

The Chromatic Dispersion of Holographic Miniprojector

Such a stereoscopic screens can be used in monochromatic light. In this case, the separation of both channels is good. In white light, however, the chromatic dispersion introduces in general a certain overlapping of images so that the perfect independent of both channels is no longer certain.

Now let us consider the chromatic dispersion of the HDS. The chromatic dispersion of the HDS is followed by the diffraction law of holographic grating.

$$nd(\sin\theta - \sin\theta') = \lambda ,\hspace{4cm}(1)$$

Here, θ-the incident angle of reconstruction beam on the screen; θ'-the exit angle of diffracted beam; d- the space of interference fringes; n- refraction index of hologram; λ-reconstruction wavelength.

The changes of output angle resulted from the wavelength changes may be obtained by differentiating equation(1)

$$\lambda = nd\cos\theta \Delta\theta ,\hspace{4cm}(2)$$

we define the changes of the output angle resulted from wavelength changes as chromatic dispersion: substituting Eq.(1) into Eq.(2), we obtain the chromatic dispersion of the HDS.

$$\Delta\theta /_{\Delta\lambda} = 2\tan\theta/_{\lambda} ,\hspace{4cm}(3)$$

Here, θ-the angle between the beam emerged from a point on the diffuser and the beam emerged from the reference point source.

It is known from Eq.(3) that the chromatic dispersion is different in the different parts of viewing zones. It is arise from changes in the different points of the HDS. In order to decreasing effect of chromatic dispersion, we use so recording geometry that the arrangements of object beam and reference beam are in a vertical plane. Then, when the screen is used, we turn the HDS through 90°. As a result, the chromatic dispersion of the HDS is vertical. In other words, there is no dispersion in the horizontal direction during observation. The dispersion will then be essentially vertical and will not effect the channels separation.

Conclusion

1. The analyses from regimes for holographic projection system is known that the single-lens projection is applicable only for small projection magnification or big screen distance. For HMP with a small screen distance and big projection magnification it is reasonable to use double-lens projection. The advantage to using double-lens holographic projector, which form zones of 3-D viewing separately for the left and right eye, lies in that it becomes unnecessary to create a viewing zone with a width not small than the interocular.

2. We have measured 3-D perception depth and the resolution of images of the BSM and the 3-D HMP. It is shown that the imaging resolution of the HMP is about 6-10 micro during higher magnification. It approximate to resolution of the BSM. The clear perception depth of 3-D images has some improvement compared to the BSM.

Therefore, due to good technical characteristics and comfortable observing conditions of the HMP, it is reasonable to make use of the HMP consisted of special HOE screen instead of the typical BSM in the product assembly and quality control of integrated circuits, printed boards and precise metals etc.

References

1. T.Okoshi, Three-Dimensional Imaging Techniques(New York, Academic press 1976).
2. J.F.Butterfield, Proc. SPIE 212 (1979).
3. Kun-xian Xu, Proc. SPIE 402(1983).
4. D.Courjon and C.Bainier, Applied Optics 21, 21, 3804(1982).
5. H.J.Caulfield ed., Handbook of Optical Holography(Academic Press, New York 1979).

Rainbow holography with a multimode laser source

F. Quercioli, G. Molesini

Istituto Nazionale di Ottica, Largo Enrico Fermi 6, 50125 Firenze, Italy

S.F. Jacobs*

Optical Sciences Center, University of Arizona, Tucson AZ 85721

Abstract

Using the coherence function of a multimode laser source, a technique is presented that produces rainbow holographic images without employing a slit for recording. A slit-shaped pupil is though synthetically produced whose extent and position can be controlled by the experimental parameters.

Introduction

Carrying out holographic work, a long coherence length of the source is greatly appreciated, as it makes the operator nearly free from care about optical path differences. However, the coherence length of even poorer sources has been sufficient in the first place to demonstrate off-axis holography: Leith and Upatnieks' first successes with plane holograms had been achieved with the 546.1 nm line of an Hg arc lamp [1].

In the case of laser sources, multimode operation degrades the coherence function according to the physics of the cavity [2]. To have an experimental appreciation of the phenomenon, a dye laser has been used where both intracavity étalon and fine tuning étalon were removed. The optical path length of the cavity was 385 mm, corresponding to a mode spacing of 390 MHz. Light from such a source has been studied with a Michelson interferometer about zero path-difference. By visual inspection of the fringe modulation in the interference pattern after displacement of a mirror in one arm, a coherence length of 0.3 mm was estimated [3].

For the purposes here under concern, such a short coherence function of a CW multimode laser source is equivalent to a short pulse duration (1 psec in the case above reported) of a pulsed laser, and can still be used for holographic work. After Nils Abramson who invented it [4,5], this technique is known as "light-in-flight holography" and it features very interesting peculiarities. Applications have already been demonstrated in the areas of single-fringe contouring, visual observation of travelling wave packets, verification of relativistic effects and more [6-10].

In this paper a further application is reported, proving the feasibility of rainbow holography without a real slit, synthesizing it instead through the source characteristics and the geometric conditions in a two-step recording process.

First step recording

As in the case of classical rainbow [11], an off-axis hologram is first recorded (Fig.1). The illuminating source is an argon laser with intracavity étalon driven at λ_1 = 514.5 nm.

For analysis purposes, a coordinate reference system (O_1,x,z) is attached to the holographic plate HP_1 with the origin O_1 about the center and the z-axis perpendicular to it. The object is in front of the plate (z>0). For the sake of simplicity, discussion will be restricted to the x,z plane only. A generic object point is so denoted by the position vector $\underline{r}_1 \equiv (x_1,z_1)$. The reference beam coming from the half-plane z>0 (transmission

* Work performed when on leave for sabbatical at Istituto Nazionale di Ottica.

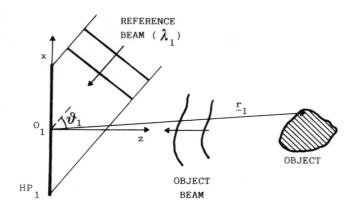

Figure 1. Step 1: Recording of a conventional off-axis hologram at plate HP_1

hologram) is a plane wave at spatial frequency $\alpha = -\sin \theta_1 / \lambda_1$. Recording is such that reconstruction, made with a plane wave at spatial frequency $\beta = \sin \theta_2 / \lambda_2$ coming from the half-plane $z<0$, causes image-to-object displacement and deformation[12]. With matrix notation the new position vector $\underline{r}_1'$ may be obtained from $\underline{r}_1$ by means of the transformation[13]

$$\underline{r}_1' = T \, \underline{r}_1 \tag{1}$$

being $\underline{r}_1, \underline{r}_1'$ column vector representations and T a square matrix defined as

$$T \equiv \begin{array}{cc} 1 & \lambda_1(\beta+\alpha) \\ 0 & \lambda_1/\lambda_2 \end{array} \tag{2}$$

Second step recording

For the second step recording a multimode laser source is used. This is a dye laser operated at $\lambda_2 = 580$ nm, the peak wavelength of R6G emission band. The coherence characteristics of that source have been mentioned in the Introduction. The plane wave at spatial frequency β illuminating HP_1 is such that a real pseudoscopic image of the object is created according to Eq. 1. Across this image a second holographic plate HP_2 is placed, parallel to HP_1 (Fig. 2). The new reference beam is at spatial frequency $\gamma = \sin \theta_3 / \lambda_2$.

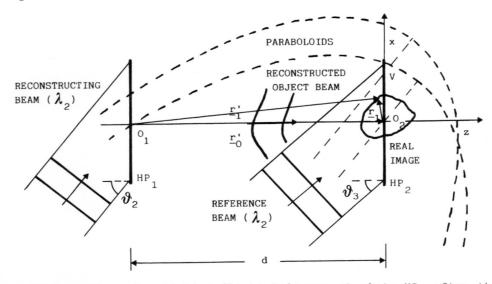

Figure 2. Step 2: Recording of a light-inflight hologram at plate HP after the real pseudoscopic image produced by HP_1

The coordinate system (O_2, x, z) is moved to the plane HP_2 by simple transfer, so that the new position vector associated to $\underline{r}'_1$ is given by

$$\underline{r}_2 = \underline{r}'_1 - \underline{r}'_0 \tag{3}$$

being $\underline{r}'_0 = T \underline{r}_0$ the position vector associated to the object's central point now used as the coordinate origin.

Recording occurs according to the particular features of light-in-flight holography. Due to the very short coherence function of the source, holographic grating buildup only works about zero path-difference between object and reference beams.

Considering a point $V(x_v, 0)$ at the plate HP_2, this may be considered the focus a paraboloidal surface with axis parallel to the illuminating beam at spatial frequency β. The intercept of such a surface with the plane plate HP_1 singles out a segment of ellipse such that rays from that segment to V all travel equal paths. These constitute the object beam. The reference beam, by means of its OPD offset, determines the actual paraboloid involved at V, and the elliptical segment on HP_1 as well. As different values of x_v correspond to different optical paths for the reference beam, a correspondence between elliptical segments on HP_1 and points along the x-axis on HP_2 is orderly stated. Experimental conditions can easily be worked out so that the above segments are well approximated by straight ones, oriented along the y direction.

Conversely, light from a single point on HP_1 is recorded on HP_2 over a segment of ellipsoid which in the same approximation is in form of a straight y-segment. The overall correspondence is so orderly stated between y-segments of HP_1 and y-segments of HP_2.

The mutual coherence condition which is the base of such correspondence is likely to travel across HP_1 and HP_2 at different speeds v_1, v_2 respectively, according to the geometrical conditions. A first-approximation approach can be made considering the distance d between the two plates in great excess of the common size $2x_{max}$ of the plates,

$$d \gg 2x_{max}.$$

Under such condition the above velocities are in the ratio

$$v_1 / v_2 = \beta / \gamma.$$

Simple geometric considerations so lead to the conclusion that a natural pole exists in the x,z plane such that the lines connecting the corresponding segments all intersect at it (Fig. 3). If the OPD offset is adjusted to make the y-segment through O_1 to correspond to the one through O_2, the pole is located along the z-axis, a distance $z_p = d/(\gamma/\beta - 1)$ from the plate HP_2.

Extension to the y coordinate shows that the pole is made of a line in the y direction. This line may be considered the effective aperture which is recorded in the second step of the process being described.

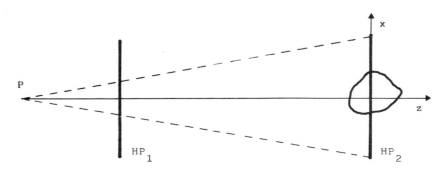

Figure 3. Formation of a synthetic slit at P in the second step recording

So far, the treatment has been carried out neglecting the short but finite extent of the source coherence length. In practice this is however a reasonable approximation, which could be made more precise taking into account the proper convolution of geometric lines and points with the actual coherence function[10].

Due to the imaging properties of the plate HP_1 where y-segments are originated, transferring to HP_2 and then to the polar line a focalization occurs at the location of the real pseudoscopic image. The y-segments so act as narrow rectangular apertures in an optical imaging system. Due to their shape, the horizontal parallax is missing.

Image formation

The plate HP_2 is illuminated with a collimated beam at spatial frequency $\delta = \sin\theta_3/\lambda_3$, conjugate as a direction to the previous beam at spatial frequency γ. So long as image formation is concerned, a coordinate transformation similar ro Eq. 1 still holds:

$$\underline{r}_2' = T' \ \underline{r}_2 \tag{4}$$

being T' the new transformation matrix

$$T' \equiv \begin{matrix} 1 & \lambda_2 \ (\delta+\gamma) \\ 0 & \lambda_3/\lambda_2 \end{matrix} \tag{5}$$

Taking into account Eqs. 1,3 the previous Eq. 4 may be written

$$\underline{r}_2' = T' \ T \ \underline{r}_1 - T' \ \underline{r}_o' \tag{6}$$

The term $T'\underline{r}_o'$ is a constant which can be set to zero with a further transfer of the coordinate system similar to Eq. 3. It clearly appears that an exact replica of the object may be obtained making $T'T = I$, being I the unit matrix. Carrying out the proper operations, this leads to the conditions

$$\lambda_3 = \lambda_1 \tag{7}$$
$$\delta + \gamma + \beta + \alpha = 0$$

Such conditions state that an undistorted image can only be recovered at a single wavelength. At the same time these suggest how to work on the parameters to obtain minimum distortion.

Considering the pole $\underline{r}_p \equiv (0,z_p)$, reconstruction occurs according to

$$\underline{r}_p' = T' \ \underline{r}_p \tag{8}$$

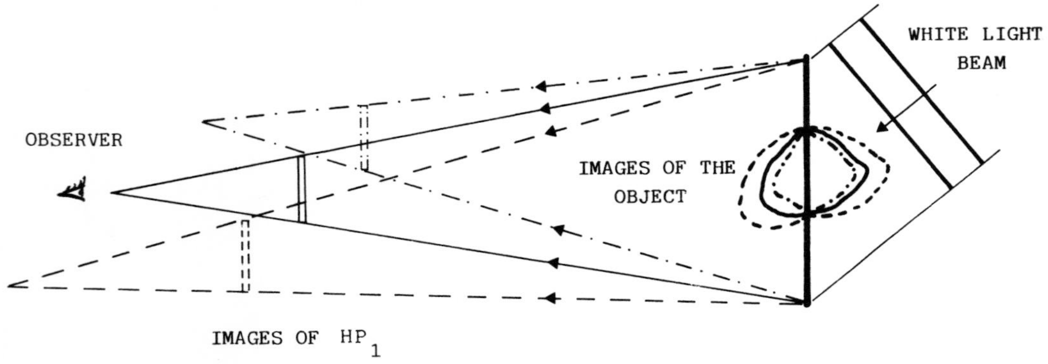

Figure 4. Holographic image formation and viewing at the synthetic slit after white-light illumination

roper operations, this leads to

$$x'_p = \lambda_2 \, (\delta+\gamma) \; z_p$$

$$z'_p = \frac{\lambda_3}{\lambda_2} \; z_p \tag{9}$$

e coordinates of the intercept between the line-image of the pole line and
This line-image extends in y direction and defines a synthetic rectangular
alent to the slit used by Benton, such that looking through it the observer
t from the whole set of plate segments. A monochrome full reconstruction is

Turni. hite light, the effect of a variable λ_3 is considered. For this purpose the explicit exp. sions for γ δ are taken into account, and a power series expansion of Eqs. 9 as a function of $\Delta\lambda = \lambda_3 - \lambda_2$ is given:

$$x'_p = z_p \sin \theta_3 \; \frac{\Delta\lambda}{\lambda_2}$$

$$z'_p = z_p \frac{\Delta\lambda}{\lambda_2} + z_p \tag{10}$$

Elimination of $\Delta\lambda/\lambda_2$ provides the locus of the pole-images in the x,z plane:

$$z'_p = - \frac{1}{\sin\theta_3} \; x'_p + z_p \tag{11}$$

The pole-images are thus aligned on a straight line of angular coefficient $-1/\sin \theta_3$, linearly dispersed as a function of the percent separation $\Delta\lambda /\lambda_2$ according to Eqs.(10).

Introducing again the y coordinate, the pole-images are turned into y line-images at different wavelengths. The observer's eye placed behind selects the actual line-image acting as the effective pupil of the system (Fig. 4). The final reconstruction is so provided in single color, which varies in a rainbow manner as the eye moves along the line of the pole-images.

Experimental results

With the technique above described a hologram has been recorded at β = 1260 lines/mm, γ= 1520 lines/mm, d = 28 cm. After reconstruction in monochromatic light, the predicted focusing effect at the polar line-image has been observed with z_p = 155 cm (the expexted value was 147 cm). A picture of that reconstruction is shown in Fig. 5, where the effect of minor periodicities in the coherence function is also visible in form of sidebands. The lines are actually bent, so pointing out the approximations introduced in the mathematical treatment.

Placing a camera at the location of that line, a picture of the image was taken as shown in Fig. 6. The all scene is visible. Observation in white light still confirmed the expected rainbow effect that made the presentation very similar to classical Benton's holographic imagery.

Conclusions

A new technique for rainbow holography is theoretically described and experimentally demonstrated. Analysis is carried out making use of simplifying approximations, which can be easily met by controlling the configuration parameters. The overall process may be regarded as a combination of Abramson's light-in-flight approach with Benton's rainbow holography. The slit however is not material but synthetically produced through a peculiar recording mechanism. The slit position can still be controlled by means of the configuration parameters.

Special care has to be taken during the second step recording, not to fog the plate with light ineffective with respect to holographic grating buildup. However, taking advantage of the nonlinear behavior of the holographic medium at the toe of the H-D curve [14], a proper

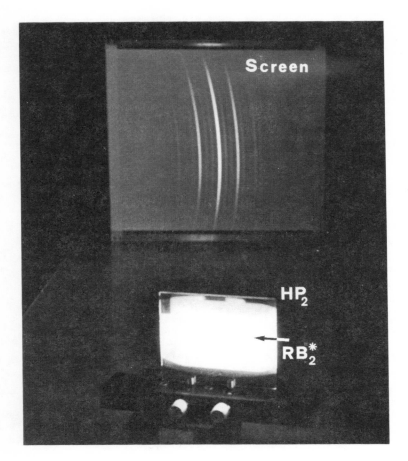

Figure 5. Focusing properties of the
final hologram illuminated
with monochromatic beam
RB_2^* (conjugate reference
beam). The screen is
located at the synthetic
slit.

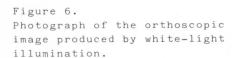

Figure 6.
Photograph of the orthoscopic
image produced by white-light
illumination.

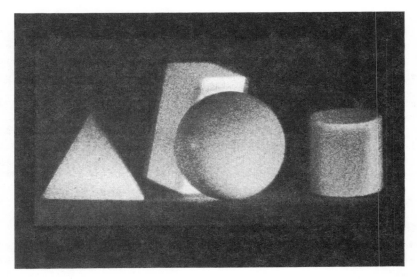

working point may be chosen so that the recording of the interference pattern is enhanced
over the bias background.

The results here presented are mainly due to the coherence function of the source, which
has been worsened with respect to usual operation. It still remains to investigate up to
which point the source characteristics can be degraded but being capable of holographic
recording.

Acknowledgments

The authors wish to thank the Amministrazione Provinciale di Firenze for partial support.

References

1. E.N. Leith and J. Upatnieks, "Reconstructed Wavefronts and Communication Theory", Appl. Opt. 52, 1123-1130 (1962).

2. H. Kogelnik and T. Li, "Laser Beams and Resonators", Appl. Opt. 5, 1550-1567 (1966).

3. F. Quercioli and G. Molesini, "White Light-in-Flight Holography", Appl. Opt. (to be published).

4. N. Abramson, "The Holo-Diagram. VI: Practical Device in Coherent Optics", Appl. Opt. 11, 2562-2571 (1972).

5. N. Abramson, "Light-in-Flight Recording by Holography", Opt. Lett. 3, 121-123 (1978).

6. N. Abramson, "Light-in-Flight Recording: High-Speed Holographic Motion Pictures of Ultrafast Phenomena", Appl. Opt. 22, 215-232 (1983).

7. N. Abramson, "Light-in-Flight Recording. 2: Compensation for the Limited Speed of Light Used for Observation", Appl. Opt. 23, 1481-1492 (1984).

8. N. Abramson, "Light-in-Flight Recording. 3: Compensation for Optical Relativistic Effects", Appl. Opt. 23, 4007-4014 (1984).

9. R. Salazar et G. Tribillon, "Synthèse d'Impulsions Subpicosecondes et Visualisation Holographique", Opt. Comm. 45, 26-29 (1983).

10. F. Quercioli,G. Molesini and S.F. Jacobs, "Zero Path-Difference Rainbow Holography", Opt. Lett. (to be published).

11. S.A. Benton, "Hologram Reconstructions with Extended Incoherent Sources", J. Opt. Soc. Am. 59, 1545A (1969).

12. J.W. Goodman, "Introduction to Fourier Optics", Mc Graw-Hill, New York 1968, 214-218.

13. G. Molesini and F. Quercioli, "Pseudocolor Contouring Based on Light-in-Flight Holography", J. Opt. Soc. Am. (submitted).

14. G. Molesini and F. Quercioli, "Evidence of a Coherence Function by Nonlinear Detection", Appl. Opt. 24, 927-928 (1985).

Some problems associated with Processing Agfa-Gevaert
8E75HD Sheet Film for Reflection Holography.

Pierre M. Boone

Laboratorium Soete voor Weerstand van Materialen en Lastechniek
Stress Analysis Division, State University of Gent
Sint-Pietersnieuwstraat 41, B-9000 GENT - BELGIUM

Abstract

   The holographic material Agfa 8E75HD sheet film is used in a Denisyuk-like type [1]
recording set-up, in conjunction with a pulsed ruby laser. A relatively simple production
method is outlined, attention being given to some practical problems : sensitivity,
processing, polarisation and color.

Introduction

   The interest in large size reflection holograms, both for metrological and for display
purposes, is still growing. On the other hand, the beam quality of ruby pulsed lasers
can now be manipulated to reach a level acceptable for high quality pictures. The
Denisyuk scheme is by far the most simple set-up for the recording of reflection
holograms, and can be used both for metrological purposes ("piggyback" set-up [2,3,4,5]) and
for single-shot applications as portraits. Apart from its simplicity, this set-up, where
object, sensitive material and laser are almost in-line, Figure 1, is also very
economical with light : the available energy is effectively used twice, and the viewing
angle at reconstruction is fairly large. The main drawbacks of this recording method are
the extreme high requirements for the processing and the sensitive material, and the
fact that the ratio of object to reference beam intensity can only be altered by treating
the object surface (painting). A variant on this technique will be presented.

   Phenomena involved in the processing of holograms are still not fully understood. Most
holographers apply photographic-type processing, almost everyone having his own "pet" -
developer. True holographic developers, based on the well-considered hypothesis of
holographic image formation, are not published. Probably some scientists have a lot of
knowledge about this subject, but little is given free due to mixing up scientific and
commercial interests. It is felt that this is a deplorable and unscientific situation;
we will describe a process we have used during a number of years with constant acceptable
results, although improvements are certainly possible.

Set-up

   With some remnants of earlier photographic and holographic experiences, we built a
semi-flexible set-up for the production of our holograms, Figure 2. The object is
illuminated by the direct beam through an attenuator and a diffusor (for safety
requirements) and sideways by two diffuse reflectors. The laser used is a 9 year old
JK 2000 system, giving 2 J maximal output. Originally the system was intended as a
holocamera, but it was modified through the years by addition of a second intra-cavity
etalon (to avoid contour fringes) and a spatial filter (diamond pinhole) between
oscillator and first amplifier; most of the unnecessary internal reflectors were removed
(energy monitors, reference wave pick-off) and the ruby rods were provided with a spiral
groove to surpress whispering modes ("orange peel"). Extreme care should be exercised to
keep everything clean; even then, the output lens and the front surface mirrors have to
be replaced regularly.

Processing

   Starting from preceding experimental work and experience in metrological holographic
interferometry, we investigated two reference developers : the straight pyrogallol [6] and
the metol-ascorbic acid superadditive developer [7]. It must be stressed this is a basic
process susceptible to improvements : the aim was to produce acceptable quality and to
collect information on the kinetics and the process parameters. Therefore baths of very
simple formulation were used. We feel that for our application the latter is best suited;
the influence of some additives was then looked for; the optimum composition will be given
later.

   Quality of holograms is generally described in terms of diffraction efficiency, S/N
ratio and resolution [8]. However, subjective factors also play an important role in the

judgment of the result : color accepted by the viewer, acceptability of small defects, amount of light accepted as optimal, contrast rendition etc. As it seems there is no standard at the moment, we used the ratio between the light reflected by an "absolute black" zone in the hologram (i.e. where there is no object wave) and an adjacent standard gray chart at 20 mm behind the film, measured with a simple comparison reflection densitometer, as an acceptable qualitative evaluation of the process; it can also be used for comparison between different processes.

Diffraction efficiency seems to be related to the density of the film after development, the optimum lying around D = 2.3. Of course, the output energy of the laser must be adapted to the reflection and (de)polarisation characteristics of the subject, but there seems to be a good relation between diffraction efficiency and macroscopic density, although they are basically quite different physical phenomena.

Process

Hypersensitization. The relative merits of some sensitisation techniques found in the literature (see e.g. ref.[9]) were studied; a combination of trietanolamine sensitisation and pre-exposure was found to give good results. The film is led through a Gevamatic DR2 dryer, in which a 3% TEA solution is replacing the normal water wash. This treatment allows one to increase the sensitivity (probably by the combination of three factors : the inherent amino-sensitisation; the absorption of some water : water dipping alone increases sensitivity, too [10], and washing out of some of the sensitizing dye, so the adsorbtion of the emulsion is lower, and also increases the efficiency. The influence of hypersensitisation can be seen on the diagram (curve 2, Figure 3).

The dynamic range of the image forming standing waves in reflection holography is larger than strictly necessary for adequate image formation. At the other hand, the holographic image is superimposed on a photographic one (direct reflection) that can be considered as noise; finally, double reflections (almost unavoidable, see later problems) give rise to macroscopic density variations ("wood structure") that will locally influence both color and diffraction efficiency. All those "photographic" irregularities can be alleviated by carrying out a weak and uniform white light pre-exposure, e.g. by the use of a high-quality enlarger. In Figure 3 the H & D curve for white light is given (curve 4). A uniform density of 0,4 or even slightly higher can be accepted. Influence of pre-exposure can be seen on curve 3, which is the curve used in practice.

Development. The basic developer is based on the formulation :

L-ascorbic acid	10 grams
4-aminophenol sulfate (metol)	2,5 g
Sodium carbonate, anhydrous	45 g
Sodium EDTA (Na salt of ethylene diamine tetra acetic acid)	2 g
Potassium bromide	0,5 g
Distilled water to	1 liter

This formulation can need some adjustment in function of the emulsion batch and/or the age of the material.

Temperature control is important; changes of more than 1°C must be avoided. Develop 4 minutes with constant agitation. The energy required can be derived from the diagram (curve 3) for development at 20°C. Develop maximum 3 sheets of 30 x 40 cm in 200 cc of developer, less if visible oxydation occurs. Wash in running water for about 30 seconds, then rinse in distilled water.

Bleach. The classical reversal bleach is used, without prior fixing :

Ammonium dichromate	3 g
Sulphuric acid, concentrated	1,5 cc
Distilled water to	1 liter

Bleach until clear, then keep the hologram one more minute in the bleach bath. Wash in running water.

Drying. Drying is best carried out with the help of another Gevamatic DR2, the tank being filled with a solution of 1 cc Agepon flow agent pro liter of distilled water.

Finish. Dehydrate in a stove at 70° for at least 30 minutes (also hardening the gelatin). Backing is normally done by spraying an index-matching varnish on the gelatin side and covering it with a matt black paint. Trials should be effectuated to see if the solvents do not influence the color of the result; even when using the same brand of paint, intrabatch variations occur.

Another possibility is to stick a black plastic foil to the emulsion side with a (good) laminator.

Some practical problems

Apart from the batch-to-batch variations in sensitivity that were already mentioned, a sensitivity drop can also occur when the emulsions are not kept under ideal circumstances (high temperature, high humidity). Slight adaptations to the developer can help.

Another, to my opinion more important problem is the birefringence of the support material. The polyester used up to now is optically active; by the fabrication process (hot stretching in both directions after extrusion), residual stresses are frozen in the material. This results in rotation of polarisation of the laser beam when passing through the backing, which is unavoidable when using the set-up proposed.

When the object itself is not depolarizing, this has not so much influence on the effective object/reference ratio as long as the object lies close to the hologram. What is worse is that, when the polarisation state is not uniform, there is no Brewster angle any more, so interval reflections inevitably occur and give rise to the hated "wood nerve" patterns. Stress-induced fringe patterns can also occur when the material is not handled with the necessary care and gentleness. An optically inactive carrier would probably be better (triacetate); manufacturers seem to be technically persuaded, but do not apply this theoretical knowledge in practice up to now, but there is hope.

Another practical problem is the intrabatch variation of the amount and/or quality of the agent responsible for the slight diffusion seen when looking through the unexposed sheets. This matting agent is introduced as small grains in the substrate (layer covering both sides of the polyester) before the real emulsion is coated to the support. It has a dual goal : to create some surface relief (to "minimize" the occurrence of equal thickness fringes), and mainly to regulate the humidity adsorbtion and desorbtion, so individual sheets do not stick together after a humidity excursion [11]. Unfortunately up to now the index of refraction of the grains does not perfectly match that of the host, so some diffusion occurs. In normal photography, this does not matter (cfr. the use of anti-reflex glass for protection of photographs) but in holography object points, lying far from the hologram plane, will appear smeared out or surrounded by a halo. Reducing the amount of grains reduces this effect, but gives rise to more pronounced thickness fringes; if the "matting" is completely omitted, the image is only smeared out as result of the finite size of the reconstruction source [12], but severely degraded by the fringes. It seems that the manufacturer is trying to optimize all this, probably also working on refractive index matching, but has not yet reached the optimum.

Safety aspects

The subjects are illuminated by a strongly diverging beam (diameter : 1,20 m with origin at 6 m); the subject is asked to focus at a green safety light placed at about 50 cm distance and about 30 cm out of the optical axis, this to avoid :

a) the large pupil diameters, that give a "waxy" look,
b) to keep the image of the laser source out of the macula,
c) to have the eyes focused in quite another place than the "origin" of the laser light.

A geometric optics calculation for this case (assuming the pupil diameter of 7 mm, focal length of the eye 17 mm) shows that the retinal power density is reduced by a factor of about 3000 with respect to the diffraction limit (size of Airy disc : 4,11 µm; size of image of point source at 6 m within eye focused at 50 cm : 0,225 mm). The corneal exposure to be considered is thus

$$106 \ \mu J/cm^2 \ \times \ \frac{1}{3000} = 0,035 \ \mu J/cm^2$$

safely lower than the exposure limit of $5.10^{-7} J/cm^2$ given by ANSI [14].

Nevertheless, accidents could occur if a shot were inadvertently fired when staring directly in the beam and exactly focusing at the 6.00 m origin. In case of doubt, we therefore introduce an additional diffusor between subject and hologram, with a scatter angle :

a) smaller than the angle subtended by the reconstruction source, typically 17 m rad for a halogen spot of 5 cm diameter used at 3 m.

b) larger than 3 m rad, being the minimum angle that (for a pulse duration of $25\,n$ sec) should be subtended by a "source" for accepting that source to be broad (see ref.[14], Figure 8-10).

In this case, we are well below the ANSI limits (table 8.2 of ref. [14]); the distance between diffusor and the eyes is not of importance [15].

On the other hand, we have also started experiments on animals in order to see if the ANSI exposure limits for intrabeam viewing are applicable to strongly diverging beams. Up to now, only one (albino) rabbit was used, so there is no statistical analysis possible; it was exposed, without diffusor, attenuator of film interposed, to :

6 times to the normal "holographic" dose,
3 times to a double dose,
3 times to a quadruple dose,
3 times to a eightfold dose.

No lesion was experimentally found, neither by use of a slit lamp, nor on examination of the prepared retina with scanning electron microscopy.

Discussion and conclusion

Denisyuk reflection holograms, produced with the set-up and processing described, reconstruct in bright green color, although they are made with a ruby laser, and show little or no cosmetic defects. It is not really understood what mechanisms are involved with that color shift. Development for a shorter time or exposure to density 1.5 shifts the color to longer wavelengths, but results in a lower (effective ?) efficiency and a lower image to noise ratio. A better method seems to be reswelling the gelatin in a post-process treatment, before drying, e.g. with sorbitol or triethanolamine.

Acknowledgement

This work was supported by the Belgian National Foundation for Scientific Research through grants 2900878 and 2001275, and the author also gratefully acknowledges the personal research grant placed at his disposal by the same institution. The technical skills of and the fruitful discussions with Mr. M. De Caluwé were of invaluable help.

References

1. Denisyuk, Y., Photographic reconstruction of the optical properties of an object in its own scattered field, Sov. Phys.- Dokl. 7, 543-5 (1962).
2. Boone, P., Toepassingen van koherent licht in de vervormingsanalyse, Doctoral dissertation, University of Gent, 1970, in Dutch, sorry.
3. Boone, P., The use of reflection holograms in holographic interferometry, Proceedings of the 1974 IEEE International Optical Computing Conference, Zürich 1974.
4. Boone, P. Use of reflection holograms in holographic interferometry and speckle correlation techniques for measurement of surface displacement, Optica Acta, Vol. 22 nr.7, p.579-589, 1975.
5. Neumann, D.B. and Penn, R.C., Object motion compensation using reflection holography JOSA 62, 1373 (1974).
6. Spierings, W., The pyrochrone process, Holosphere, NY, Vol. 10 nr. 7 & 8, p.1-2.
7. Ascorbic acid as developing agent was first studied by Kendall (1935); it was brought to our attention by J. Gutjahr of the Photographische Fachhochschule Köln, Germany. See also the MAA3 developer of Benton.
8. Joly, L. and Van Hoorebeeck, R., Development effects in white light reflection holography, Photographic Science and Engineering, 24, p.108-113 (1980).
9. Kodak Plates and Films for Scientific Photography, p.17-23, Eastman Kodak C°, 1973 (Standard Book nr. 0-87985-083-3).
10. Joly, L., Private communication.
11. Joly, L. and Van Hoorebeeck, R., Private communication.
12. Gutjahr, J., Die Zeit im Hologrammen, paper presented at the International Holographic '84 Meeting, Frankfurt, 1984.
14. Sliney, D. and Wolbarsht, M., Safety with Lasers and other Optical Sources, Plenum Press, NY, 1980, p.261 and following.
15. Ross, I., Considerations of Eye-Safety in intense diffuse illumination, Optics Communicatics, Vol. 12 nr. 1, 1974, p.46-50.

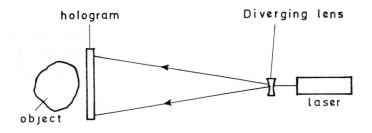

Fig:1 Denisyuk setup

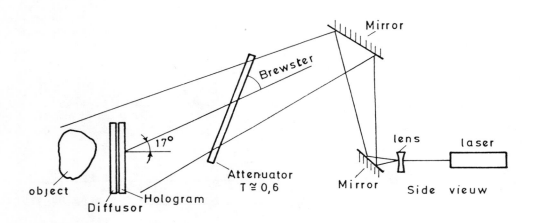

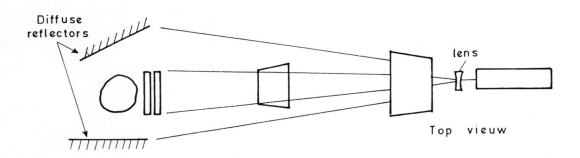

Fig:2 Modified setup

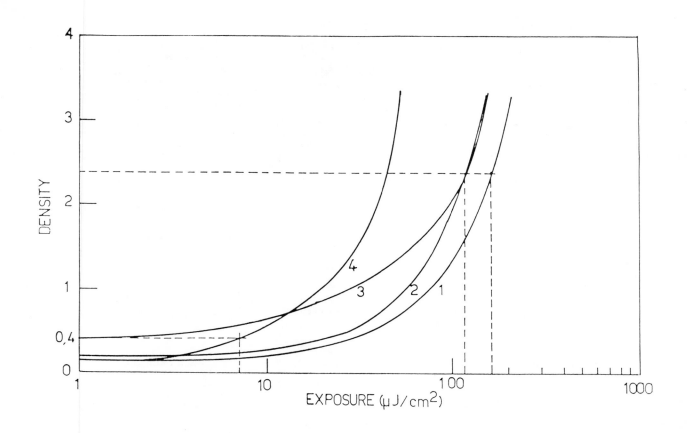

Figure 3. Caracteristic curves for Agfa-Gevaert 8E75 sheet film, processed with Ascorbic acid developer, under constant bath agitation during 4 minutes and a temperature of 20,5°C.
Curve 1, film from package; curve 2, hypersensitized film, curve 3 hypersensitized film pre-exposed with 20 lux. sec.
The wedges for these three curves are exposed with ruby laser light.
Curve 4, hypersensitized film exposed with white light. Although the exposure scale must be determined in lux. sec., for easy comparison, the values are transformed to μJ/cm². Density values of 2,3 for curves 1, 2 and 3 (optimum holographic density) and 0,4 (pre-exposure density) and the corresponding exposure energies are indicated. Values for emulsion nr. 46498026.

Wide angle distortion free holographic head-up display

J. C. Perrin

Télécommunications Radio Téléphoniques
Le Plessis Robinson, 92350, France

Abstract

A new optical design of a 60° x 30° holographic display is demonstrated. The arrangement uses two holograms, a relay lens and a Schmidt plate. The first hologram is used as collimator and combiner and gives complete see trough capability. The second hologram is a field hologram. Ray traces and spot diagrams are shown, which have been obtained with a computer program especially developed for this analysis.

Introduction

The use of holographic elements in avionic displays has been proposed many years ago[3]. Reflection hologram offers the unique advantage of permitting the fabrication of almost ideal beam splitters and combiners to project the green image of a display to the observer without affecting the visibility of the outside world. This property is obtained by suitable recording of an interference pattern in a thick phase layer of dichromated gelatin.

Several applications of such holograms has been described in the litterature. An holographic one-tube Goggle was presented by Cook in 1979[2]. In the same time, several approaches have been made to design a wide field of view head up display for avionics applications[3]. A complete analysis of the holographic combiner for the LANTIRN program was presented recently[1].

In 1979 a research program was conducted at TRT to design a wide field of view holographic display. Two applications where anticipated. One was for night vision image intensifiers equipemnt like goggles and episcops, the other for helmet mounted displays and head up displays for thermal imagers. In this article we describe our approach and present the results which we have obtained.

Geometrical properties and image quality given by an holographic collimator

Figure 1 illustrates the basic operation of an holographic collimator. The hologram H in front of the observer images the pupil of the eye (centre 0_1) on the exit pupil of a relay lens (centre 0_2). Its focal surface F is conjugated from the screen P by means of the relay lens T. The image of the screen is therefore projected at infinity to the observer. The screen can be for example the TV output of an head up display or the phosphor of an image intensifier tube. The hologram is of the reflexion type. It is produced with two coherent beams propagating in the opposite direction and having their focus points at 0_1 and 0_2 respectively. The two waves are not necesseraly spherical, but must have their focal points well defined (from the photometric point of view) in order to concentrate the energy into the area surrounding the pupils.

We have determined by computer ray traces the image quality given by the holographic collimator when the two constructing beams are spherical waves. The fringes which are recorded in the volume of the hologram are ellipsoids with focal points in 0_1 and 0_2. Our conclusions are :

1. The focal surface F of the collimator depends on the first order on the shape of the surface on which the hologram is recorded.
2. In any case the focal surface is curved and inclined to the optical axis. The distorsion is very high.
3. The geometrical aberrations in F are very high except if the number of fringes recorded in the volume of the hologram is small. This occurs when the hologram is made on an ellipsoid having its focal points in 0_1 and 0_2. In this situation, the hologram has the geometrical properties of an elliptical mirror and the photometric properties of a reflexion hologram. In such case the image is free from astigmastism.

Many attempts have been described in the litterature to optimize the shape of the two waves constructing the hologram. A great difficulty is also to design the relay lens. Because of the asymmetrical configuration of the focal surface F, the relay lens is also asymmetrical. The image quality which is obtained is poor, and in any case the amount of distorsion is unacceptable for most applications.

The best configuration is described in reference 1. The aberration are reduced by decreasing the distance $0_1 - 0_2$. The hologram tends to a spherical mirror with the pupil located near its center. Such a reflective collimator gives an image and no distorsion in a wide field of view. But the design includes two supplementary holograms operating as plane mirrors to transfer the focal surface out of the observer space.

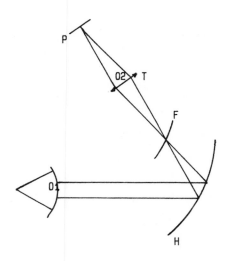

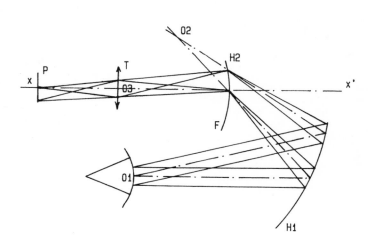

Figure 1. Basic operation of the holographic collimator

Figure 2. Proposed configuration

Our approach is different (figure 2). We propose to use two holograms H_1 and H_2. H_1 is the collimator with focal surface F.
H_2 is a field hologram superimposed to the focal surface F of the collimator. H_2 conjugates the exit pupil 0_2 of the collimator and the pupil 0_3 of the relay lens. On this way, the relay lens is rotationnaly symmetric, having its axis xx' in coïncidence with the main axis of symmetry of F. This configuration greatly simplify the optical design of the relay lens and leads to reduced distorsion.

Optical Design

The best configuration of the hologram H_1 with almost zero distorsion is obtained with a classical spherical mirror (figure 3).

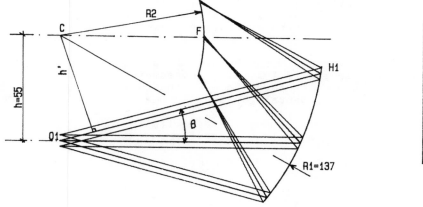

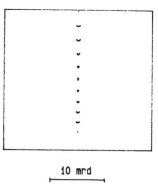

Figure 3. Spherical mirror used as a collimator

Figure 4. Spot diagram in F

With the pupil excentered of h from the center C of the mirror, the focal surface F is a sphere with radius $R_2 = h/\sin\left[2 \operatorname{asn}\left(h/R_1\right)\right]$.

The focal length of this collimator is given by $f = R_2$. The distorsion is practically zero :

- horizontally, the focal length is constant for any field of view because 0_1C is axis of revolution,
- vertically, for the direction θ, we have $h' = h \cos \theta$ and $f' = \dfrac{h \cos \theta}{\sin [2 \text{ asn } (\frac{h \cos \theta}{R_1})]}$.

With $\theta < 15°$, we have $f' \# f$. The distorsion in the vertical direction is also very small. Nevertheless, the image quality is quite poor. For practical reasons, the distance h of the pupil from the main axis must be great enough to remove the focal surface from the vertical field of view. It results to a large amount of spherical aberration in the image, as shown by the spot diagram on figure 4. The spot diagram was obtained with a pupil diameter of 6 mm. The resolution, of the order of 25 mrd, is not acceptable.

The classical method to remove the spherical aberration of the spherical mirror is to use a Schmidt plate in the pupil of the mirror. Here only an excentered portion of the plate would be used, corresponding to the size of the pupil of the eye. Nevertheless, this correcting element would also greatly affect the direct vision through the hologram H_1. Moreover, the introduction of this element in immediate proximity of the eye is not recommended. The prefered solution has therefore been to put the correcting Schmidt plate in the pupil 0_3 of the relay lens. This leads to the overall design shown on figure 5.

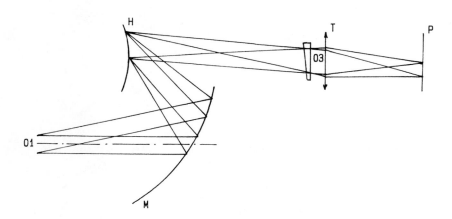

Figure 5. Complete optical set up

- M is an holographic spherical mirror. It is equivalent to a spherical mirror coated with an holographic thick film. Its pupil is located in 0_1 on the eye of the observer. The reflectivity of the hologram for the green light of the phosphor P is about 90 %, and its transmission for the light coming from the outside world is of the same order of value. This makes the holographic coating very valuable, as this result would doubtfully be obtained by classical thin film technology. We describe thereafter how this hologram can be made.

- H is the second hologram used as a field hologram. H can be as well a reflection hologram as shown on this figure or a transmission hologram as initially represented on figure 2. The solution using a reflection hologram has been prefered in our final design because it affords a better mechanical implementation of the overall optical scheme in the space volume available.
On the optical point of view, H conjugates the pupil 0_1 of the eye with the pupil 0_3 of the relay lens T. The method for producing H is also described thereafter.

- T is the relay lens which transfers the image of the phosphor P into the field hologram H. In the pupil of T is placed an excentered Schmidt plate to compensate for the spherical aberration of M.

On this basis a complete design has been evaluated (figure 6).

The optical parameters are :

- Field of view : horizontally   60°
                  vertically   30°
- Focal length : 24,25 mm
- Image diameter :   28 mm
- Focal length of the collimator : 74,79 mm

- Magnification of the relay : 3,08
- Maximum pupil diameter : 8,5 mm

These parameters correspond for example to an helmet mounted head up display. The image can be the screen of a mini TV tube, or the fiberplate of a third generation image intensifier. In our initial design, an existing relay lens was selected, having a real pupil in the image space with sufficient distance from the rear glass to permit the introduction of the Schmidt plate. This lens was not optimized for our design. It is normally used with a much larger image distance.
Nevertheless, it was prefered because of its availability. As the image field hologram is curved in the opposite direction from the normal Petzval curvature of the lens, it has been necessary to curve also the object to compensate for the field curvature. In practice this can be obtained with a fiberoptic plate whose one face is plane an the other curved.

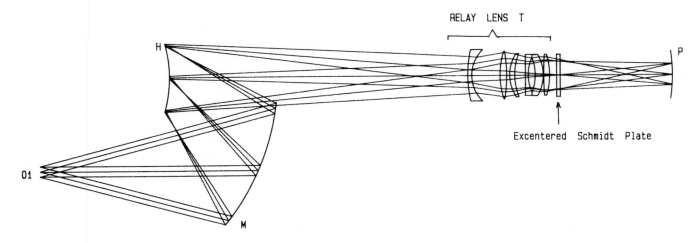

Figure 6.   Ray traces of our final solution

In order to optimize the Schmidt plate and determine the image quality, a computer program has been written on a desktop computer. This proprietary program uses the classical ray trace routine for spherical and aspherical surfaces and mirrors which is routinely used in our laboratory for optical design. A special option was added to take into account the diffraction law given by holographic elements. The kind of hologram considered in this program is general, that is that both the reference and object waves which are used to construct the hologram can be produced by any optical scheme including mirrors and lenses. Nevertheless the program accepts only one hologram of this type. For this reason, the spherical hologram H_1 was calculated as a spherical mirror. Only the field hologram was considered as an hologram from the mathematical point of view. The optical scheme to construct this hologram is described farther on.
Using this program, the Schmidt plate was determined in order to obtain the best quality at the centre of the field. A sixth order plate was used with equation :

$$x = a\,y^2 + b\,y^4 + c\,y^6$$

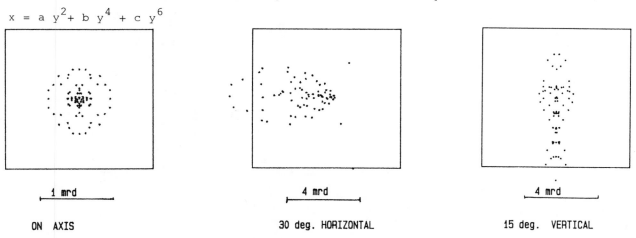

Figure 7.   Horizontal and vertical spot diagrams

The figure 7 shows the spot diagram obtained for a 60° x 30° field of view and a 6 mm pupil diameter.
On axis, the image quality is satisfactory. The spherical aberration of the collimator is almost completely removed.
At 30° horizontally, the degradation of the image is significant. This can be attributed to the relay lens which was not optimized for this magnification.
At $\pm$ 15° vertically, the figure shows some residue of astigmatism. This is due to the spherical collimator whose vertical field of view is limited.
In conclusion, the image quality of the design is acceptable in the 30° x 60° field of view. Nevertheless, the overall resolution could be significantly improved by using another relay lens especially designed for this purpose. This is particularly true for the horizontal field of view. Vertically the image quality is more limited by the collimator.

Hologram Fabrication

Holographic Collimator

The spherical collimator can be coated using conventionnal thin film technology or using holographic recording in dichromated gelatin. The advantage of the holographic technology is to reflect a narrow hand of wavelength very efficiently as well as offering complete see-trough capability. This advantage result from the bragg effect in the thick gelatine and is obtained only if the recording geometry of the hologram is compatible with the position of the pupils.

The proposed procedure to record the hologram satisfy this condition. In a first step, a reference Hologram H_R is made using the configuration shown on figure 8.a. H_R records the wave reflected by the spherical mirror M when illuminated by a diverging point source 0_1 and using a plane reference wave π_1. In this first operation, M is a purely reflecting mirror and 0_1 is located at the centre of the pupil. The wave which is recorded by H_R is highly aberrant, with a paraxial focus at 0_2.
The holographic coating on the spherical combiner is made in the second step shown on figure 8.b. Using the same arrangement as on figure 8.a, the spherical mirror is replaced by the combiner, the internal face of which has been coated with dichromated gelatin. The object and reference waves for producing the reflection hologram are identical to the waves procuded on figure 8.a, but propagating in the opposite direction :

- The object wave is spherical converging at 0_1
- The reference wave is restituted by H_R using a reference plane wave π_2 identical to π_1 but propagating in the opposite direction.

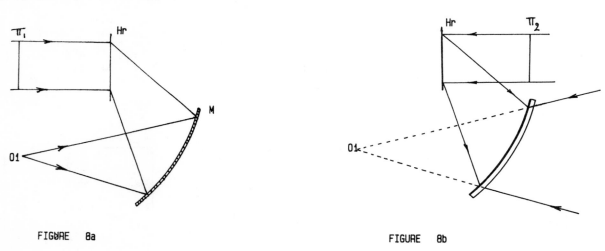

FIGURE 8a

FIGURE 8b

Figure 8. Fabrication of the holographic Collimator

Both waves interfere in the gelatin to produce an interference pattern which is recorded as index modulation in the gelatin. Only one fringe is spherical of centre C. The other fringe pattern on both sides of these central fringe is slightly distorted and will produce the highest bragg effect for a pupil location in 0_1.
The spherical combiner which is obtained on this manner transmit the outside world without attenuation at collimates the display to the observer with almost 90 % photometric efficiency.

Field Hologram

The fabrication of the field hologram is more conventionnal.
The function of this hologram is to give a well defined image in 0_3 of the entrance pupil
0_1 (figure 5). This condition is necessary to obtain a sharp image of the pupil on the
Schmidt plate and have the best image correction in the whole field of view.
We have simulated on the computer the situation in which the field hologram is only stigma-
tic between 0_2 and 0_3. In this case the hologram is made with two spherical waves having
their focal points at 0_2 and 0_3. In this situation the image in 0_3 of the entrance pupil 0_1
is highly aberrated. For this reason, the correction of the aberrations obtained with the
Schmidt plate is less efficient. In practice , we have determined that the horizontal field
of view can hardly exceed 10°.

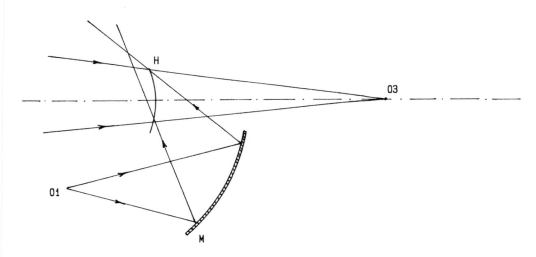

Figure 9. Fabrication of the field hologram

The arrangement to record the field hologram is shown on figure 9. The reference wave i.
obtained with a diverging point source located at 0_1. After reflection on the spherical
mirror M, this wave illuminates the hologram.
The object wave is only a spherical wave converging in 0_3. On this configuration, a reflec
tion hologram is produced. The same arrangement could be used to make a transmission
element by using a diverging object wave.

The computer evaluation described above has been made in accordance to this recording
arrangement. For this reason, the program takes into account the situation in which both
object and reference waves are produced using conventionnal optical lenses and mirrors.

Conclusions

A reflection type holographic head up display has been described with a 60° x 30° field
of view and no distorsion. Optimisation of the system has been achieved using computer ray
traces and the image quality given by the spot diagrams is shown.
The design could find applications for avionics head up displays or for helmet mounted
displays.

References

1. C.H. Vallance. The approach to optical system designs for aircraft head up displays.
SPIE. PROC. Optical System design analysis and production, Genève, 1983.
2. L.G. Cook. Systems Engineering of an advanced Holographic One-tube Goggle.
PROC. SPIE. 23 RD international Symposium and instrument display, San Diego, 1979.
3. Head up Display. Concept under development Aviation week, May 1977.

PROGRESS IN HOLOGRAPHIC APPLICATIONS

Volume 600

Poster Session

Progress in holographic cinematography

P. Smigielski[*], H. Fagot, F. Albe

Franco-German Research Institute Saint-Louis (ISL)
68301 Saint-Louis, France

Abstract

Two important progresses were achieved for the first time: 1) recording of single exposure cineholograms of living bodies on a 126-mm film, at a frequency of 25 holograms per
second. Limitations of 3-D movies by holography are described. 2) recording of double-exposure cineholograms of reflecting objects, a loudspeaker membrane and the vertex cranii of a
bald-headed man. These experiments show the interest of interferometric cineholography for
industrial applications.

Introduction

Holography is expected to become a potential tool for achieving in a near future scientific three-dimensional cinematography which will be observable without wearing glasses.
The first holographic[1] film in Western Europe called "Holotrain" was recorded in October
1983 on a 35-mm film at a taking rate of 24 holograms per second[**]. Thereafter, two important progresses were achieved for the first time: use of a 126-mm film and recording of
holographic films by double-exposure of non-transparent phenomena. The four dimensions of
space-time are from now available at a laboratory level. This means that decisive step
forward can be made in both the investigation and the better understanding of physical
phenomena. An outlook on the future, especially in view of a large audience for 3-D movies,
will be given. Finally the possible scientific uses will be evoked.

Holography and stereoscopy

The principal difference between the conventional techniques used for both the recording
and reconstruction of three-dimensional objects or phenomena (stereoscopy) and the holographic methods is essentially due to the manner in which the information is recorded. Stereoscopy is characterized in that two images of the object are recorded on a photographic
plate or film using photographic lenses. In the case of holography, luminous interferences
are recorded on the photographic plate without imaging the object. To generate these interferences the light wave scattered from a laser illuminated object and a reference wave
coming from the same laser, but which does not strike the object, are superimposed with one
another (principle of holography). In both cases, however, the final analysis of the information in view of the visual perception is made in the same way, that is with the aid of
the eyes and the brain. But only holography allows the three-dimensional nature to be entirely reproduced. If the structure is observed with one eye only, 3-D effect vanishes in
stereoscopy. This is not the case in holography. The hologram, or the holographic film in
the case of holographic cinematography, behaves like a window which is open to the scene.
Any displacement in front of the window allows the point of sight to be changed at will
such that objects masked by obstacles can be perceived as if they were really present
(parallax effect). Presently this advantage is however counterbalanced by a serious drawback
which should not be neglected, that is holographic recording calls for the use of a
laser[***]so that recording of holograms is limited to small scenes (a few m³). In effect
the difference between the optical paths taken by object and reference beams must be below
the coherence length of the laser which, in turn, is related to the length of the wave
trains emanating from the laser. Thus, if the coherence length is equal to 2 m (case of a
high-performance pulse laser[****]), the depth of the scene will not exceed 2 m. Further it
is difficult to protect the hologram from the ambient direct light so that holograms cannot
always be taken on the outside.In the case of stereoscopy, the point of sight cannot be selected at will. In effect it is determined in the recording step. But the major drawback
inherent in stereoscopy stems from the fact that the spectators must wear special glasses

----

[*]   Also professor at Université Louis Pasteur, Strasbourg
[**]   For the activities conducted in view of achieving this scientific first run, Pro-
       fessor P. Smigielski was awarded the Alfred Kastler prize 1985 by the "European
       Photonic Association, Research Group from the Parliamentary Assembly of the Council
       of Europe"
[***] Another important drawback for entertainment purpose: the film actors must protect
       their eyes from the intense laser light with special glasses, as shown in the
       picture 3
[****]   for an interference fringes contrast equal to 0.3

(polarizing spectacles or coloured spectacles, or spectacles having a fast shutter action) in order to be capable of distinguishing between the two images of the object, each of them being thereby seen by the left or the right eye. This is no doubt the reason why stereoscopy has not found widespread use in movie theaters.

Holographic recording of objects scattering light by reflection (holography by reflection)

Holographic recording of transparent objects (holography by transmission)

Holography is well known to have allowed the complete visualization of three-dimensional phenomena and/or structures. For many years efforts have been made to apply this method to cinematography (the term "cineholography" was introduced as early as 1965[2]), but it has been only recently that the first significant experiments were performed: 1976 in the Soviet Union[3], 1981 in the United States[4], and 1983 in France[1]. The preliminary experiments conducted in France and concerned with the motion synthesis should also be mentioned here[5]. Now the question arises as to the reason why cineholography has come so late into practical use? To answer this question, we must distinguish between two methods of holographic recording: holographic recording of objects scattering light by reflection (also termed "holography by reflection") and holographic recording of transparent objects (also termed "holography by transmission")[*]). As its name implies, holography by reflection is characterized in that the waves scattered as a result of the reflection of the illuminating wave by the object are recorded. This means that the surface of the object is visualized. In contrast, in the holographic method of recording transparent objects (holography by transmission), only the shadows of the objects are visualized and not the objects themselves. Consequently, it is practically the whole energy of the illuminating wave, which strikes the film when transparent objects are investigated (air flows, shock waves, plasmas,...). In the case of the reflection technique, only an extremely small part, a few thousandths of the quantity of light emanating from the laser, arrive on the hologram. The holographic recording of objects scattering light by reflection is therefore seen to need a laser with a high energy output. In contrast holographic recording of transparent objects can be done with a laser having a relatively low energy output. Moreover no high coherence is required. These are the reasons why holographic cinematography based on the recording of transparent objects made its way rapidly in the scientific domain. In effect lasers with features such as a very high repetition rate, low energy and slight coherence have always been available. Inversely holographic cinematography based on the recording of objects scattering light by reflection, that is a real 3-D motion picture technique accessible to a large audience, has been achieved only recently. In fact this technique calls for the use of lasers delivering 24 or more high-energy pulses per second and having a high coherence. Those lasers were available at some laboratories and at ISL. Thus fifteen years after the first ISL cinematographic hologram of a phase object (shock waves had been recorded[6], the first West European holographic film based on the reflection technique could be achieved[1] with the aid of a laser designed and built at ISL by H. FAGOT with the cooperation of A. HIRTH. This film is a small step forward to 3-D cinematography having a high repetition rate which is particularly suitable for scientific applications.

Current state of the art in research

In all the aforementioned experiments, the separation of the images on the film (35 mm or 70 mm) is achieved in a conventional way, i.e., via the translational motion of the film by means of the feed system of a conventional cinema projector, the optical components of which have been removed. More recently a continuous film-transport camera (OMERA) which can be operated with film ranging from 16 to 126 mm was especially adapted to our experiment. The continuous run of the films is a very classical technique used in high-speed cinematography or holography. Each hologram is exposed with a pulse of the laser. The synchronization of the laser repetition rate with the feed rate of the film allows a series of jointed holograms to be obtained on the film. The film can run continuously because the exposure time involved is only of the order of 15 ns. In effect, in order to obtain holograms of a good quality, the film must not cover a distance, during the exposure time, which exceeds one tenth of the wavelength of the light beam. This leads to a tolerable maximum feed rate of approximately 3 m/s whereas the feed rate of a conventional 70-mm film equals 1.2 m/s. Furthermore, in contrast to conventional cinematography, the intermittent film motion is not mandatory.

----

[*]) This terminology is different from the classical one used mainly in the field of artistic holography: reflection holography means that the reference light source and the observer are on the same side (Denisyuk set-up)

V.G. KOMAR conducted the first experiments in this field of interest (1976)[3]. He succeeded in making observable to several persons the holographic picture thanks to a holographic screen which allowed the 3-D nature of the pictures to be preserved*)[4]. The light source used for forming the holograms was a ruby laser (emitting in the red). Thus the picture frequency (24 Hz) could only be attained by using a great number of lasers. It seems that KOMAR has recorded a 70-mm film at 8 Hz using 8 lasers! Experiments conducted in the United States (DECKER, 1981)[4] allowed the picture frequency of 20 Hz to be attained with the aid of a frequency-doubled Nd:YAG laser (green light). Because of the limited energy per pulse (7 mJ), however the scene recorded on a 70-mm film was very small. The object filmed was a small figure ("SNOOPY") of some cms placed on a plate which rotated with a speed of 1 r.p.s.. The experiments conducted at ISL (1983) were similar to those performed by DECKER. But the scenes recorded were relatively more large (m³). This results from the fact that the pulse YAG-laser used at ISL had a relatively more high energy output (30 mJ per pulse). Further, we recorded for the first time double-exposure holographic films of non-transparent objects (time-reflecting objects).

New experiments conducted at ISL

1. Recording on 126 mm-films[8]

The holographic arrangement used at ISL was a conventional one. A small part of the illuminating wave is used to form the reference beam which illuminates directly the film. By superimposing approximately equally the light beam scattered from the scene with the reference beam, microinterferences are generated on a 126-mm film. The latter has a high resolution and is sensitive to the green light (wavelength $\lambda = 0.532$ μm). The green light is obtained after the infrared beam of light ($\lambda = 1.06$ μm) emitted from the YAG laser has gone through a frequency-doubling crystal with an efficiency within 20 to 40%. After the photographic development the film is solely illuminated with the reference beam. This occurs in the same way as in the recording step, but the laser used is not necessarily the same. Normally a cw-laser is used (ionized argon laser) operated at a wavelength which approaches that of the recording laser ($\lambda = 0.514$ μm $\approx \lambda = 0.532$ μm) to avoid geometrical aberrations[9]. By using a Helium-Neon red laser the image quality is however good enough. It is shown mathematically that with respect to the film and in the direction of the scene recorded, the reconstructed light wave has the same amplitude and phase as that emitted from the scene in the recording process. If one is placed behind the film, it is possible to perceive part of the light wave with one eye or with the two eyes provided the film is sufficiently wide (it is the case here)**). This means that the scene is seen as if it were really present. It can be photographed at different points of sight and with different adjustments, if necessary. This has been done in order to illustrate the results achieved (fig.1, 2). Several sequences entitled "Holomobile" and "Christiane et les holobulles"("Christiane and the holo-bubbles") were recorded, for the first time at a taking rate of 25 holograms per second. This rate allows easy video recording of the reconstructed images. The good stability of the coherence of the YAG laser allows to record 30 m length film without problems. "Holomobile" shows the tumbles of a toy car (and its image in a plane mirror) in a 50 cm square wood box (fig. 1, 2). "Christiane et les holobulles" exhibits a young lady who produces soap bubbles and projects them in the direction of the observer (fig.3, 4).

2. Interferometric cineholography[10]

In May 1985 our YAG laser has allowed for the first time to record holographic films by double-exposure of non-transparent phenomena using a conventional 35-mm camera specially adapted for holographic recording.
- "Holoparleur" (holo-loudspeaker) shows the deformation and displacements of a loudspeaker diaphragm of 25 cm in diameter vibrating at frequencies of 20 Hz and 70 Hz (fig. 5, 6).
- "Holocrâne" (holo-skull) visualizes "in vivo" the vertex cranii of a bald-headed man (fig. 7, 8).
    In both cases the double-pulse of the coherent beam of light required for the holographic interferometry is generated under the action of two successive pumpings of the same YAG laser. The laser and the camera were operated at a frequency of 10 Hz. The time interval separating two pulses was 4 and 10 ms. Thus the sensitivity of this dynamic interferometric arrangement is increased.

----

*) This screen is a holographic optical element giving several separated images (4 in the soviet experiment) from one object. A serious drawback: the brightness of each image decreases as the number of superimposed holograms on the same photographic plate increases[7]

**) The 126 film allows in the reconstruction process to have a stereo picture of the scene by direct viewing without wearing special glasses.

Outlook on the future

The objective of the research activities conducted at ISL is to achieve 3-D cinematography by holography with a high repetition rate in order to investigate dynamic non-transparent phenomena encountered in physics.

1. Single-exposure cineholography

The technique of cineholography as described in this paper will meet the demands made by the scientists. This is not the case, however, for entertainment cinematography (3-D movies). The use of pulse lasers for taking pictures leads to serious drawbacks:
- the depth of the scenes is limited to a few meters,
- the film actors must protect their eyes from the intense laser light,
- the velocity of the objects under recording must be very low; 1 m/s in the direction of the camera with a pulse duration of 20 ns.
- full-color cineholography cannot be envisaged within a foreseeable period even if it is theoretically possible (many things are theoretically possible).

Problems are also encountered in the reconstruction process performed either with lasers (presence of a "speckle" in the reconstructed images) or in white light (reduction in the depth of the scene). The main problem is the visualization of the film by many people:
- the use of reflecting holographic screen is theoretically possible (see the KOMAR experiment[3]). But, as said above, there are some serious drawbacks.
- one can use a film larger than 126 mm. Why not 1 meter? But, how many people can watch such a film in the same time ?

It seems that cineholography for entertainment purposes (3-D movies) will stay a very long time either a funny curiosity to see in museum or a prestige advertizing. A solution to the problem inherent in 3-D cinematography would be to use holography not for the recording step, but only in the reconstruction process, as this is the case for multiplex holograms[10], for instance. Then, holography would be the strongest candidate tomorrow in the field of 3-D movies, because it might enable the spectators to observe the 3-D nature of the scene without wearing glasses. Moreover spectators might change their point of sight by simple motion!

2. Double-exposure cineholography

The combined use of interferometry and cineholography is of a great interest for the 4-D investigation of physical events varying with time such as the deformations of materials and structures. In particular the aeronautical industry is interested in this technique which is expected to allow non-destructive testing of materials in quasi real time.

With one YAG laser working at a low repetition rate (10 Hz), the method is recommanded for the investigation of deformations and/or vibrations occurring at low or very low frequencies in the fields of mechanics, physiology or heat events. But by using two YAG lasers with their beams well superimposed, the time interval separating the two pulses can be chosen at will and the study of quasi-steady objects vibrating at all frequencies is possible.

References

1. Smigielski, P., Fagot, H., Albe, F., Cinéholographie. Congrès OPTO 84, Paris, 15-17 May 1984, ICO-13 congress, Sapporo, Japan, Aug. 20-24, 1984. 16th Int. Congress on High-Speed Phot., Strasbourg, 27-31 August 1984. Optical Metrology, NATO Workshop, Viana Do Castelo, Portugal, July 16-27, 1984. La Recherche n° 163, February 1985
2. Paques, H., Smigielski, P., Cinéholographie, C.R. Acad. Sc. Paris, 260, 6562, 1965
3. Komar, V.G., Principle of the holographic cinematography; 1st European Congress on Optics Applied to Metrology, Strasbourg, 1977
4. Decker, A.J., Holographic cinematography of time-reflecting and time-varying phase objects using a Nd:YAG laser. Optics Letters, vol. 7, n° 3, March 1983
5. Aebischer, N., Bainier, C., Multicolor holography of animated scenes by motion synthesis using a multiplexing technique, SPIE Congress: 3-D Imaging, Geneva, April 21-22 1983
6. Smigielski, P., Hirth, A., New holographic studies of high-speed phenomena, 9th Int. Congress on High-Speed Photography, Denver, Col., August 1970
7. Royer, H., Smigielski, P., Expositions multiples sur un hologramme. Qualité des images restituées. Applications. Symposium on applications of coherent light, Firenze, Sept. 1968
8. Smigielski, P., Application of holography to non-destructive testing. Colloquium "Horizons de l'Optique 85", Besançon, May 31, 1985, and Cineholography . "Holopro 85" Belfort, 20-21 Juin, 1985

9. Vienot, J.Ch., Smigielski, P., Royer, H., Holographie optique, développements, applications. Dunod éd. , Paris, 1971

10. Fagot, H., Cinéholographie interférométrique. Colloque Holopro 85, Belfort, 20-21 Juin 1985

11. De Bitetto, D.J., Holographic panoramic stereograms synthetized from white light recording. Appl. Optics, 8, n° 8, 1969

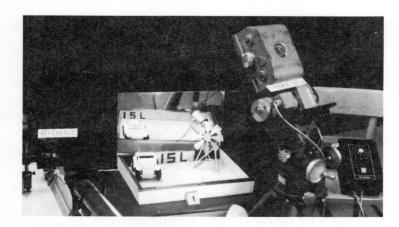

Fig. 1: "Holomobile" recording set-up with a 126-mm camera

Fig. 2: Pictures taken from the 126-mm holographic film "holomobile"

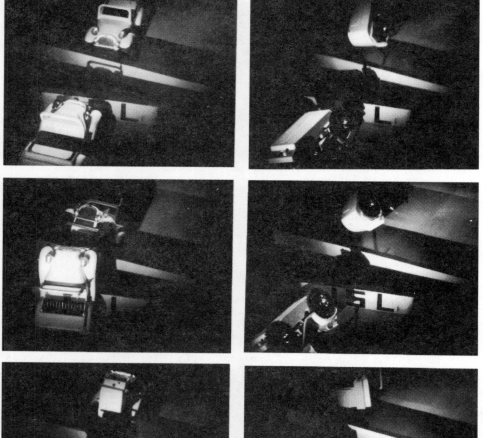

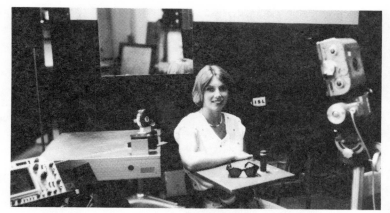

Fig. 3: "Christiane et les holobulles":
before the recording

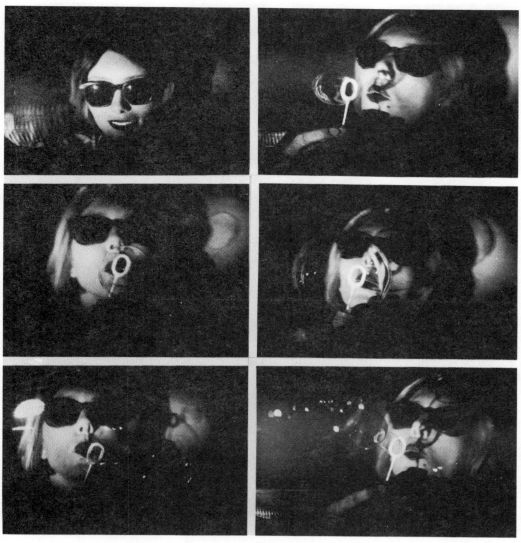

Fig. 4: Pictures taken from the 126-mm holofilm "Christiane
et les holobulles"

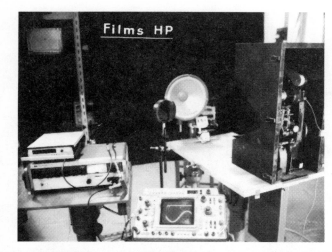

Fig. 5: "Holoparleur": recording
arrangement with the
35-mm camera

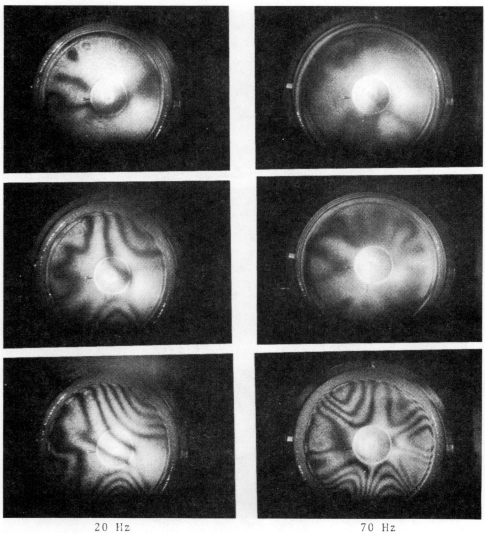

20 Hz   70 Hz

Fig. 6: Reconstructed images taken from the 35-mm holofilm
"Holoparleur". Weakly excited loudspeaker.
Double-exposure 2 × 10 Hz, Δt = 4 ms

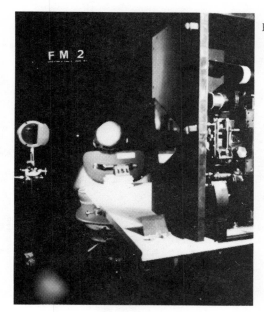

Fig. 7: "Holocrâne": view of the bald head and
35-mm camera before holographic recording

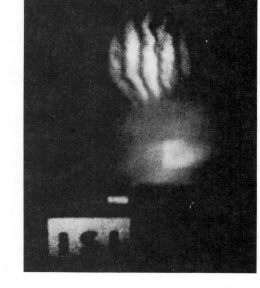

Fig. 8: Pictures taken from the 35-mm
film "Holocrâne". Steady living
head. Double-exposure 2 × 10 Hz,
Δt = 10 ms

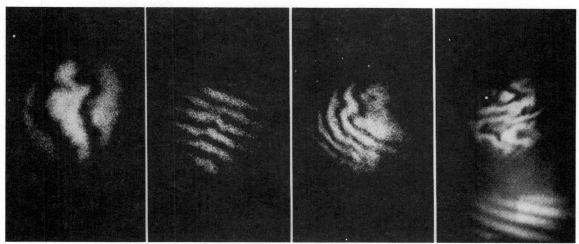

A new method for compensating and measuring any motion of 3D-objects in holographic interferometry: recent developments

A. Stimpfling - P. Smigielski*

Franco-German Research Institute of Saint-Louis (ISL)
68301 Saint-Louis, France

Abstract

Up to now holographic interferometry did not allow the study of an object motion generating too many interference fringes. Our method is general and resolves this problem in all cases. This paper gives some new developments and applications of this technique.

Introduction

The use of holographic interferometry is only possible if the interference fringe pattern due to the optical path variations remains readable. As a consequence, the object displacement (or deformation) must be small enough. In general this condition is not fulfilled in non-destructive testing or in mechanical studies, for example. Therefore it is necessary to develop a method which allows the detection of defects in structures or in materials and the measurement of 3D-displacements in industrial environment.

The existing methods (double-reference beam by SURGET[1], sandwich holography by ABRAMSON[2]) do not apply to a general displacement (of any amplitude).

The method we propose[3,4] is really a general method allowing the compensation and the measurement of the complex motion of an object the amplitude of which can be greater than the coherence length of the laser used for the holographic recording.

This method is called "CMC": Complete Motion Compensation in holographic interferometry. It can be used for real-time, time-average and double-exposure holographic interferometry even in the case of high-speed phenomena.

"CMC" applied to real-time holographic interferometry

1. Principle (fig. 1)

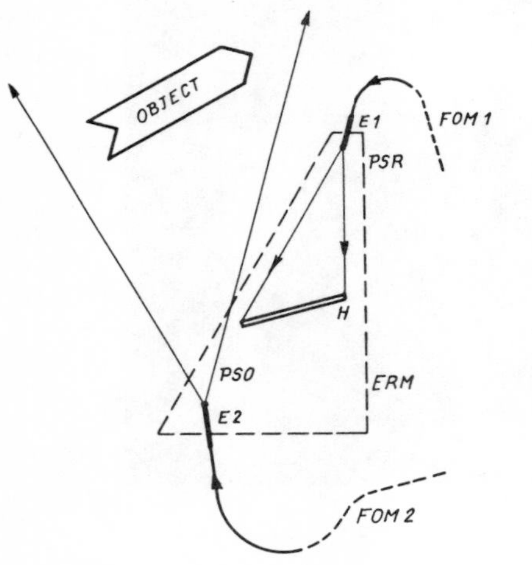

The rigid block ERM composed by the holographic image and by the illuminating object beam is moved to exactly superimpose the object and its holographic image (infinite fringe i.e. exact compensation of the optical path variations). This involves that the reference point source (PSR) and the object-point source (PSO) are rigidly connected to the hologram H. Two monomode optical fibers FOM_1 and FOM_2 connected to the rigid block ERM via the rigid connectors E_1 and E_2 are used to conduct the laser light respectively towards the object and the hologram. A set of mirrors driven by a computer can be used instead of optical fibers to eliminate problems arising from the use of pulse lasers.

A perfect optical path compensation only occurs for rigid body motion. In the case of the deformation of an object, the compensation can be done only for a small area. The whole object surface deformation can be studied spot by spot. In both cases rigid displacements and deformations can be quantified by measuring the displacements of the whole rigid block ERM without taking account of the fringe spacing or localization distances, as is normally done in classical holographic interferometry.

Figure 1. Motion compensation in real-time holographic interferometry

Consequences:

- It is possible to determine the sign of the local displacement, thus one hologram is enough to yield the location of the "hollows and humps".
- The "CMC" method allows the comparison between a reflecting object and a reference reflec-

*) also professor at Louis Pasteur University, Strasbourg

ting surface.
- Real-time interferometry allows the study of vibrating objects subjected to continuous displacements of any amplitude.

2. Assisted repositioning

If the interference fringes generated by the displacement or the deformation of the object are too close to be detected or if the object and its holographic image are not superimposed, it is first of all necessary to adjust the holographic picture on the object until exploitable fringes are obtained. One process consists in observing fine cracks or marks on the object surface with the aid of a binocular microscope. Another process uses one or more holographic interferometers in directed light. One or more small mirrors are set on the object, reflecting the illuminating object beam in the direction of one or more small areas that have been reserved for this purpose on the hologram. The setting of this or these interferometers to obtain the infinite fringe is easy and leads to the automatic adjustment of the holographic image. It is also possible to use a method of speckle interferometry[4].

3. Use of a computer to move the rigid block ERM

The complexity and the precision of the holographic image displacements require a computer-aided displacement of the rigid block ERM (fig. 1). Six degrees of freedom must be obtained with the help of motorized translation devices (0,1 µm step by step). The system designed and built by the French Company "MICROCONTROLE" and adapted to our holographic experiment is shown at figure 2 and figure 3.

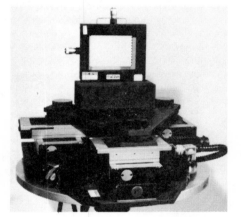

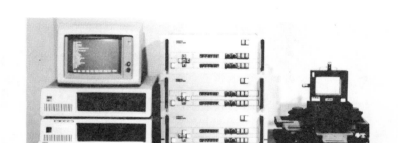

Figure 3. Overall view of the hologram displacement set-up

Figure 2. Motorized hologram carrier

Computer   Driving elec-   Motorized holo-
                tronics   gram carrier

4. Applications

Some feasibility experiments have been achieved to demonstrate the interest of the "CMC" method:
- detection of a defect (non-destructive testing). A screw generates a local micrometric deformation of an aluminium alloy plate 14 cm × 22 cm in size. This simulated defect is well visualized in spite of great amplitude rigid displacements of the plate (fig. 4, 5).

Figure 4. Front
view of the sam-
ple. On its left
side are fixed
the components
of the inter-
ferometer help-
ing the "CMC"

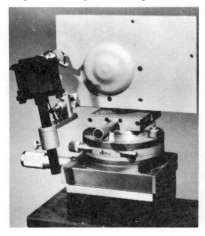

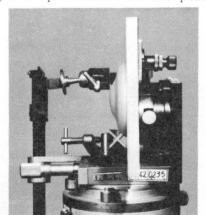

Figure 5. Side-
view of the sam-
ple. The micro-
metric screw
used for local
distortion is
visible on the
right

- clamping of a beam in a vice. Figure 6 shows the interference fringes obtained after clamping. Fringes appear on all parts of the set-up. On the beam itself they are too close to be visualized. Pictures 8 to 10 show the compensation of the rigid motion achieved successively on various parts of the mechanical set-up. The "CMC" applied to the beam itself shows three fringes due to the clamping (fig. 11).

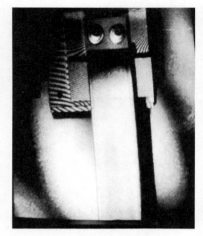

Figure 6. Real time: the beam is clamped in the vice

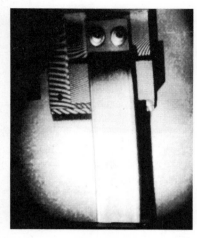

Figure 7. Real time: "CMC" on the base plate

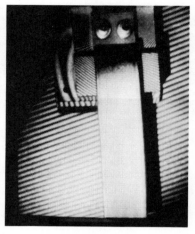

Figure 8. Real time: "CMC" on the translation unit

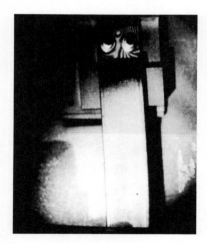

Figure 9. Real time: "CMC" on the working jaw

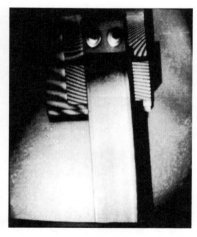

Figure 10. Real time: "CMC" on the static jaw

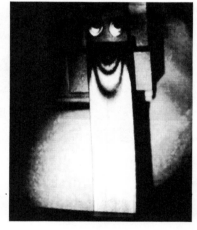

Figure 11. Real time: "CMC" on the beam

- deformation of a beam due to local tooling. The hologram of the metallic beam is recorded before tooling. After tooling (fig. 12), the beam is set again in the original holographic arrangement. Local compensation is easily made on different parts of the beam (fig. 13 to 16) showing deformations due to the tooling.

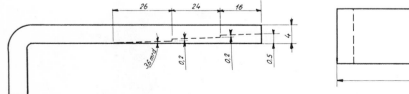
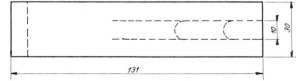

Figure 12. Description of the beam tooling

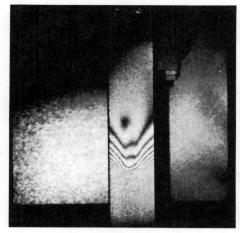

Figure 13.   Real time: "CMC" on
the undistorted part
of the beam

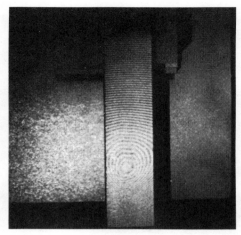

Figure 14.   Real time of the beam

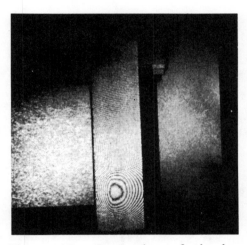

Figure 15.   Real time of the beam

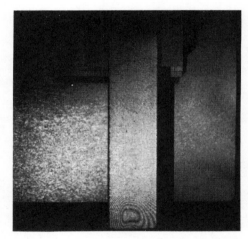

Figure 16.   Real time of the beam

"CMC" applied to time-average holographic interferometry

The "CMC" technique can be used to record a hologram of a vibrating object subjected to a rigid displacement[4].

"CMC" applied to double-exposure holographic interferometry[3]

To maintain the advantages of the principle explained above, the two exposures are recorded on two separate holographic plates: the first exposure is made on a photographic plate SH_1, then the second exposure is made on another plate SH_2 located behind the first one (fig. 17).

Figure 17.   Optical arrangement for motion
compensation in double-exposure
holographic interferometry

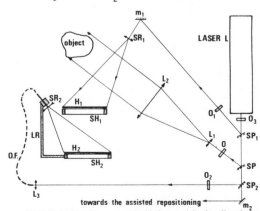

In the case of a rigid motion of the object, if one of these two holograms has its reference point (SR$_2$) rigidly connected to the photographic plate (SH$_2$), it is possible, during the reconstruction, to compensate up to the infinite fringe the optical path variation due to object translations (collimated object beam) (fig. 18 to 20). However, a local compensation can be achieved for a general displacement. Therefore, the method can be used for non-destructive testing.

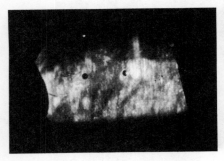 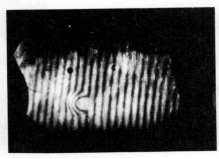 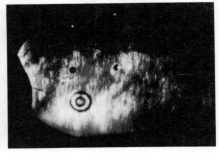

Figure 18. Double-exposure. Translation of 1 mm: the fringes are not visible

Figure 19. Double-exposure. Partial "CMC"

Figure 20. Double-exposure. Exact "CMC": the local distortion is well visible

Nota: A special optical arrangement allows the study of an object simultaneously subjected to translations and to a rotation: the collimated object beam must be parallel to the axis of rotation of the object.

Conclusion

The "Complete Motion Compensation in holographic interferometry" appears as a powerful tool not only for qualitative evaluation (non-destructive testing) but also for quantitative studies (displacement and deformation measurements). A special arrangement allows the study of rotating objects. Moreover, this new technique can be used to analyse dynamic or high-speed phenomena.

References

1. J. Surget, International Conference on Applications of Holography, Jerusalem, August, 22-26, 1976
2. N. Abramson, Conference on the Engineering Uses of Coherent Optics, Strathclyde University, Glasgow, April 1975
3. A. Stimpfling, P. Smigielski, OPTO 84 Congress, Paris, May 1984, ICO-13 Congress, Sapporo, Japan, August 1984. Optical Engineering, vol. 24, No. 5, Sept.-Oct. 1985
4. A. Stimpfling, Thesis, Louis Pasteur University, Strasbourg, Oct. 1985

Use of an endoscope for optical fiber holography*)

F. Albe, H. Fagot, P. Smigielski

Franco-German Research Institute Saint-Louis (ISL)
68301 Saint-Louis, France

Abstract

The problems of recording holograms through optical fibers are discussed. A holographic arrangement is tested; it is composed of:
- a c.w.- or pulse-laser,
- one or several multimode fibers and an imaging fiber bundle for the object beam,
- a monomode fiber for the reference beam.

Various holograms of a small object were recorded and some reconstructed images are shown.

Introduction

Holography is increasingly used in industry for non-destructive testing of materials[1]. In an industrial environment, however, the object to be investigated is not always easily accessible.

The use of optical fibers in the holographic arrangement allows to overcome this difficulty[2-15].

In a first stage we tested a holographic arrangement with fibers but without endoscopic element[16-18]. After that we introduced an imaging fiber bundle between the object and the holographic plate.

Below we describe:

1. the difficulties involved with the general use of optical fibers in holography,
2. holographic experiments conducted with c.w.-laser,
3. holographic experiments conducted with pulse laser.

Problems arising from the use of optical fibers in holography

The problems encountered in recording holograms through optical fibers as well as the difficulties involved with the development of interferometric fiber sensors are of the same nature. However both techniques work under opposite conditions.

Interferometric fiber sensors have found a widespread use. A detailed description of these components can be found in Refs.[19-21]. Nevertheless their principle of operation should be briefly recalled herein.

Interference fringe pattern is generated by two coherent beams of light emanating from the same laser and traveling through optical fibers. One of the fibers, called the sensing fiber, is exposed to the variations of a physical parameter and the phase of the guided light beam is modulated. The other fiber, called the reference fiber, is not exposed to these variations. The interference fringe pattern moves. The shifting process is analysed by means of a photodetector and a suitable demodulator is employed to calculate the original variations of the physical parameter. In order to insure a good sensitivity, strong fringe shifting should be obtained with the slightest possible variation in the physical parameter to be measured.

The holographic technique is characterized as follows: the interference fringes generated by both an object-illuminating beam of light and a beam of light called reference beam are recorded in a photosensitive material.

In contrast to the method based on the use of transducers, the fringes forming the hologram must have a great stability. This requirement must be met at least in the exposure procedure of the photosensitive material. There are two possible ways for obtaining a good stability:

----

*) This work was supported in part by the DRET (Paris)

1) Care must be taken to avoid any variation of the physical parameters (such as temperature, pressure, electromagnetic field, vibrations, shifting, twist, mechanical strain,
   etc...) capable to act on the phase or on the polarization of the light beam transmitted by the fiber when c.w.-lasers are used which need relatively long recording times.
   It is therefore of advantage to protect the fibers with suitable coverings, to fix them
   adequately without mechanical strain, and to avoid any effect due to air flows, etc...

2) The exposure time must be as short as possible in order to "freeze" the effects produced
   by the aforementioned events. This means that a pulsed laser must be used. Unfortunately
   other problems are to be faced in this case, which must be related to the high power
   density of the emission of light attained for injecting the very strong laser pulses into
   the fiber. Thus 100 mJ delivered in 20 ns would lead to a power density equalling 60
   megawatts/cm^2 in a 100 μm-diameter fiber. Problems are therefore encountered not only on
   the entrance face of the fiber, but also in the fiber itself. In pulse laser holography
   without fibers, focussing of the light beams must be avoided at all events. In general
   the beams of light must be made to converge in order to have them injected into the
   fiber. Air may be ionized and a breakdown may occur on the entrance face of the fiber or
   in its immediate vicinity. This will result in a loss of energy and in a possible deterioration of the entrance face of the fiber. Moreover the fiber itself will be exposed
   to the risk of cracking. Finally non-linearity events may arise[22] which lead to a
   decrease in the coherence length and/or to frequency shifting of the light wave.

   In the experiments reported in the following sections, attemps were made to record
holograms in the presence of the aforementioned phenomena. The experimental set-up is
shown in picture 1. It is composed of:

- a c.w.- or pulse-laser as light source;
- a multimode fiber (diameter = 1 mm, length ≈ 1 m) to illuminate the object;
- a microscope objective associated to an imaging fiber bundle made by Olympus (80 000
  fibers of 10 μm, length = 1 m) placed between the object and the holographic plate;
- a polarization-preserving, single-mode fiber (diameter = 5 μm, length ≈ 2 m) in the reference beam.

   The faces of the fiber bundle are square (4 mm × 4 mm) and the resolution in incoherent
light is 15 μm.

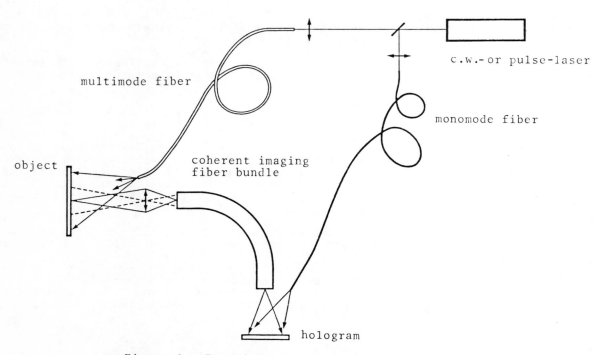

Figure 1 - Experimental set-up

Experiments conducted with c.w.-lasers

The light source was a Kr$^+$ (500 mW, 6471 Å) or Ar$^+$ (2 W, 5146 Å) laser. We tested the following types of holograms:

    1> single exposure
    2> double exposure
    3> real time
    4> time average.

For the cases 1, 2 and 3 the object was a part of a metallic plate; with a lens magnification of 1/5 the square field investigated had 2 cm side-length. For the last case the object was a vibrating round (diameter 2 cm) or square (side = 2 cm) plate.

Figure 2 shows two examples of deformations detected by double-exposure holography.

Figure 3 shows three examples of photographies obtained in real-time experimentation.

Figure 4 shows three examples of time-average holography.

In real time experimentation we used the technique described in ref.[23,24]. The principle of this method involves a rigid connection of the reference point source to the hologram.

The most difficult experiment is the real-time holography. When the superposing of the reconstructed image on the object is realized it is necessary to immobilize the imaging fiber bundle. Both faces being immobilized, a very small displacement of the bundle destroys the interference system. The other fibers, i.e. the illuminating fiber and the reference beam fiber, can be moved without destruction of the interference system.

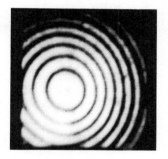
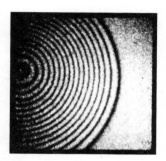

a> deformation of 2,2 μm (Kr$^+$ laser)   b> deformation of 4,2 μm (Ar$^+$ laser)

Figure 2 - Double exposure holography

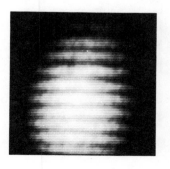
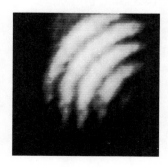
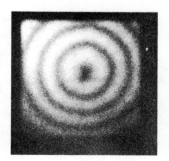

a> rotation of 25 seconds   b> deformation of 1,5 μm   c> deformation of 1 μm
   around an horizontal axis

Figure 3 - Real time holography with Ar$^+$ laser

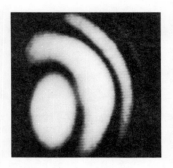
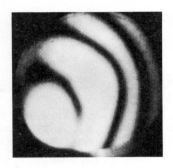
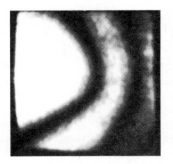

a> vibration at 2700 Hz of   b> vibration at 3700 Hz of   c> vibration at 2750 Hz of
   a round plate   a round plate   a square plate

Figure 4 - Time-average holography with Ar$^+$ laser

Experiments conducted with pulse laser

The light source was a frequency-doubled YAG-laser. It delivers pulses of 30 mJ in 20 ns at 5320 Å. This laser was used in our laboratory to record cineholograms[25-27].

The object was also the metallic plate used in c.w. laser experimentation. Single- and double-exposure holograms were recorded.

Figure 5 shows an example of a reconstructed image of a single-mode hologram and fig. 6 shows three examples of reconstructed images of double-exposure holograms: in fig. 6a a rotation of 25 seconds around a vertical axis was detected and 4 μm and 1,5 μm deformations of the object were detected in the case of fig. 6b and 6c, respectively.

Figure - 5 Single-exposure
holography with YAG-laser

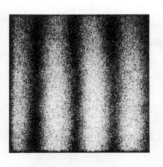
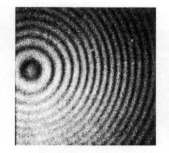
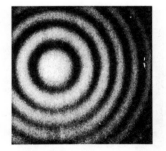

a> rotation of 10" around a   b> deformation of 4 μm   c> deformation of 1,5 μm
   vertical axis

Figure 6 - Double-exposure holography with YAG-laser

Conclusion

This experimental set-up realizes a holographic endoscope. It will be used for investigating deformations or visualizing defects in mechanical structures.

References

1. Smigielski, P., General review on the investigations conducted at ISL in the field of holographic non destructive testing. Conference on industrial applications of holography non-destructive testing Brussels, May 3-5, 1983, - SPIE vol. 349

2. Caufield, H.J., Harris, J.L., Light pipe holography. Applied Optics vol. 6, n° 7, July 1967

3. Hadbawnik, D., Holographische Endoskopie. Optik 45 (1976), Nr. 1, 21-38

4. Yamamoto, U.,Precise measurement by holography: Holography combined of fiber optics. Rapport interne, Université de Tokyo (1978)

5. A.M.P.P. Leite, Optical fiber illuminators for holography, Optics Communications, vol. 28, No. 3, March 1979

6. Wüthrich, A., Lukosz, W., Holography with guided optical waves, Applied Physics by Springer-Verlag 1980, 21, 55-64

7. Motoki Yonemura et al., Endoscopic hologram interferometry using fiber optics, Appl. Optics, 20.9. 1 May 1981 pp. 1664-67

8. Gilbert, J.A., Herrick J.W., Holographic displacement analysis with multimode-fiber optics, Experimental Mechanics pp. 315/320, August 1981

9. Herriau, J.P., et al., Optique cohérente en temps réel sur cristal électrooptique BSO, Rap. interne du Lab. Central de Recherches de Thomson CSF, déc. 1981

10. G. von Bally, Otoscopic investigations by holographic interferometry: A fiber endoscopic approach using a pulsed ruby laser system. In Optics in Biomedical Sciences Proc. of the Int. Conf. Graz, Austria, Sept. 7-11, 81, Springer Series in Optical Sciences No. 31 - Springer Verlag Berlin, Heidelberg, New York

11. Gilbert,et al., The monomode fiber. A new tool for holographic interferometry, Experimental Mechanics, vol. 23, No. 2, June 1983

12. Bouteyre, Le Floch, Introduction des fibres optiques en holographie, Rapport interne de l'Aérospatiale, Etablissement d'Aquitaine, Saint-Médard en Jalles, 1983

13. von Bally, G., Gradient index optical systems in holographic endoscopy, Applied Optics, vol. 23 No. 11, 1 June 1984

14. Bjelkagen, Hans I., Pulsed fiber holography: a new technique for hologram interferometry, Optical Engineering, July-August 1985, vol. 24, No. 4

15. Dudderard, T.D. and Gilbert, J.A., Real time holographic interferometry through fiber Optics. J. Phys. E Sc. Instr. vol. 18, 1985

16. Albe, F., Utilisation des fibres optiques en holographie, ISL - R 102/83

17. Albe, F., Holographie ultra-rapide par fibres optiques. J. Optics 84, vol. 15, n° 6

18. Albe, F., Fagot, H., Smigielski, P., Use of optical fibers in pulsed holography, European Conf. on Optics, Oct. 9-12, 1984, Amsterdam - SPIE, vol. 491

19. Pocholle, J.P., Tardy, A., Mesures de grandeurs physiques fondées sur l'utilisation des fibres optiques. Conférence européenne d'optique 1980, Horizons de l'Optique 80, Pont-à-Mousson, 22-25 avril 1980

20. Giallorenzi, T.G., et al., Optical fiber sensor technology. IEEE Transaction on microwave theory and technique, vol. 30, No. 4, April 1982

21. Arditty, A., et al., Les capteurs à fibre optique: principes et technologies, Actes du congrès OPTO 82, 16-18 nov. 1982, Paris, ESI Publications

22. Stolen, R.H., Non-linearity in fiber transmission, Proc. of the IEEE, vol. 68, No. 10, Oct. 1980

23. Stimpfling, A., Smigielski, P., New method for compensating and measuring any motion of three-dimensional objects in holographic interferometry. Optical Engineering, Sept.-Oct. 1985, vol. 24 No. 5

24. Stimpfling, A., Nouvelle méthode de correction et de mesure des déplacements quelconques d'un objet tridimensionnel en interférométrie holographique. Thèse de doctorat d'université, U.L.P., Strasbourg, 12 oct. 85

25. Smigielski, P., et col., Cinéholographie. Actes du congrès Opto 84, Paris, ESI Publications

26. Smigielski, P., Fagot, H., Albe, F., Three dimensional cinematography by means of holography. Conférence Horizons de l'Optique, Besançon, mai 85

27. Fagot, H., Cinéholographie interférométrique, colloque holopro 85, Belfort, 20-21 juin 1985.

Design for a commercial application of a holographic scanning system

Charles C. K. Cheng

Research & Development Division, Lockheed Missiles & Space Company, Inc.
Palo Alto, California 94304

Abstract

A simple, low-cost, versatile holographic scanning system was developed for use with dichromated gelatin holograms or similar high-quality copies made by hologram techniques. The fabrication of the disk holographic scanner is described in detail. The optical configurations of several high-density scan patterns were generated, and they are applicable to commercial scanning requirements.

Introduction

Traditionally, it has taken too long and cost too much to convert basic data into a form that can be immediately processed by a computer. Technology is now strengthening the data-entry link with a variety of new microelectronic-based products. One of the most significant developments is the laser-scanner-equipped supermarket point-of-sale (POS) system designed to read the universal product code (UPC) on grocery items. The scanning POS system speeds the checkout process and reduces error. Furthermore, the system can provide ways to improve overall store operating efficiency, e.g., in inventory control, reordering, and labor scheduling.

Today, there are laser scanners operating at 12,600 supermarket sites.[1] The recent increase in the number of scanner installations has been caused above all by the reduced cost of the scanner. Previously, the cost of a laser scanner was higher than that of an electronic cash register. Through a cost-effective program at NCR Corporation's Cambridge facilities, we looked into the feasibility of using a holographic scanning technique to replace some of the high-cost components such as polygons, mirrors, and lenses. This work resulted in simplification of manufacture and assembly. Consequently, the laser scanner has gained general commercial acceptance.

We successfully fabricated several multihologram disk scanners in Kodak holographic plates (type 120-02) and made high-quality copies in dichromated gelatin, obtaining high diffraction efficiencies. Figure 1 presents a photograph of the fabricated scanning disks (master and copy). Figures 2 and 3 show the basic laser UPC scanner function diagrams. Holographic scanners are not only a satisfactory replacement for many mechanical scanners such as the rotating polygon, but offer the following important advantages:

1. The optical arrangement can be simpler because of the diffracting and imaging functions of holograms.
2. Tolerances for wobble can be larger because the diffraction angle depends primarily on the spatial frequency of the hologram (this is only true for the transmission hologram, however).
3. Less air turbulence in the gas surrounding the scanner and less stress differentials within the body of the scanner will yield higher resolution.
4. Rotational speed can be lowered without sacrificing scan distance, since the scanning angle of holographic scanners is independent of the number of hologram facets on the scanner.
5. Production cost per unit can be lower.
6. When the holographic scanner is used for receiving the laser light scattered from the UPC symbol, it can act as a spectral filter to separate the laser light from the ambient light.

These combined advantages make holographic scanning one of the most promising candidates for future effective UPC scanners.

There are several areas in which holographic optics have interesting properties: (1) they can be recorded on curved surfaces, since their properties are primarily determined by the recording wavefronts, while the properties of conventional optics are determined by the shapes of the surfaces; (2) several holographic optical elements can be recorded at a single location in a hologram plate; (3) holographic optics can be designed and fabricated to operate outside the visible spectrum - the design of such holographic optics generally requires the aberration balancing and wavelength compensation techniques

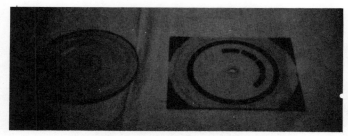

Figure 1. Photograph of holographic scanning disks (master at left, copy at right).

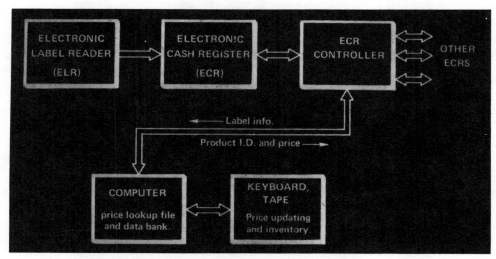

Figure 2. Laser UPC scanner attachment and the electronic cash register system.

available in a computer program; (4) aspheric hologram lenses can be easily fabricated with a combination of cylindrical and spherical wavefronts, or distorted wavefronts.

Principles of holographic scanners

Since the first proposal of a holographic scanner was made by I. Cindrich,[3] a number of papers[4-9] and several patents[10-13] have appeared on various holographic scanners. Also, laser scanning techniques developed over the past decade have been well implemented by supermarket scanners and laser-based electronic printers.

The basic principle of holographic scanners is to change the spatial frequency component of a hologram in a scanning direction. For the present application of holographic scanners to the POS systems, the rotational mode is more convenient in many respects. We will discuss principles of various rotational holographic scanners.

As shown in Fig. 4, the direction of scan lines is determined by the position of the incident laser beam with respect to the center of scanner disk. The distance L_s scanned by a hologram is given by

$$L_s = [F(\sin\theta_d) + d] \cdot \theta_r \qquad (1)$$

where θ_d is the diffracted angle of the center ray of the laser beam, d is the distance between the center of the scanner disk and the center of the hologram, and θ_r is the angular size of the hologram.

The spot size of a laser beam focused by a holographic lens is determined by the F-number of the holographic lens, as well as the shape of the incident laser beam. In this aspect, holographic optics are similar to conventional refractive optics, i.e., conventional lenses. Aberrations produced by a holographic lens are strongly dependent on the wavelength and illuminating angle of the incident laser beam. If the wavelength and illuminating angles of the incident laser beam are the same as those of the reference beam used for constructing the holographic lens, there are no aberrations. Several authors have discussed in detail the aberrations of holographic optics.[14-15]

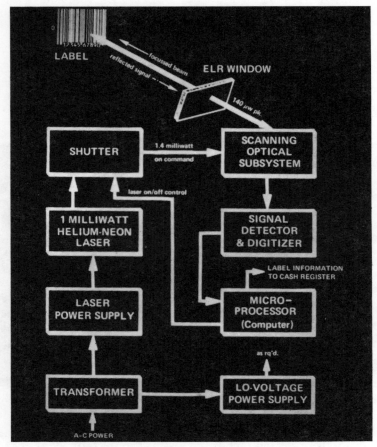

Figure 3.   Basic laser UPC scanner functions.

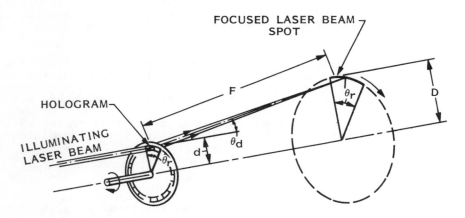

Figure 4.   Holographic scanning of laser beam.

Fabrication of disk holographic scanners

To demonstrate the feasibility of the holographic scanner concept as applied to the POS systems, we first fabricated several multiholofacet scanners in Kodak holographic plates and then copied them into dichromated gelatin plates to increase the diffraction efficiency of the holograms. The multihologram scanner has 28 holograms, of which 24 holograms recorded on the outer circumference of the scanner disk are for the vertical scan lines and 4 holograms recorded on the inner circumference are for the horizontal scan lines. If dichromated gelatin is sensitized to a wavelength of 0.6328 μm, holograms can be directly recorded in a dichromated gelatin plate.

By using a F-number of 250 and measuring the size of an unexpanded laser beam, we can determine the required focal length of the holographic lens. Since the diameter of our He-Ne laser was 2.34 mm at the $1/e^2$ power points, the focal length of the holographic lens should be 527 mm. If necessary, however, we can change the focal length of the holographic lens, since the size of the laser beam can be modified by the optical system.

Next, we will determine the position of the point source with respect to the enter of the holographic scanner disk (Fig. 5). Since the maximum angular size of θ_r of the hologram for a vertical scan line of 76.2 mm is /12 rad, the distance D between the point source and the center of the scanner disk should satisfy the following conditions:

$$D = F \sin \theta_d + d \, \frac{7.62}{\pi/12} \tag{2}$$

or

$$\theta_d > \sin^{-1}[(29.1 - d)/52.7] \tag{3}$$

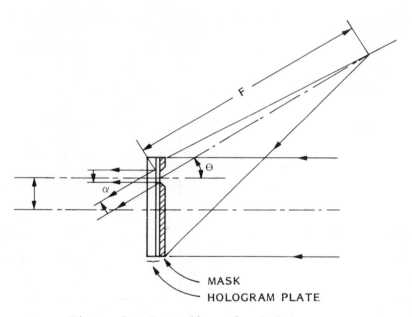

Figure 5. Recording of a hologram.

Construction of holographic scanners

Using the design parameters stated in the previous section, we set up the hologram recording system shown in Fig. 6. This shows the mask used for recording holograms. First, we recorded the 24 holograms on the outer circumference of the holographic scanner disk necessary for 24 vertical scan lines. The recording procedures were as follows:

1. Expose the first hologram at the position 0.
2. Rotate the hologram plate by 15° ($\pi/12$ rad).
3. Move the hologram-mask assembly 6.35 mm to a new position (along the line that is perpendicular to the object beam).
4. Repeat steps 1-3 until all 24 exposures are completed.

Similarly, we recorded four holograms on the inner circumference for the horizontal scan lines. This time, the first exposure started at the position L. Between exposures, the hologram plate was rotated by 35°, and the hologram-mask assembly was translated by 19.5 mm.

The exposed plate was developed by using Kodak standard development procedures. The developed holograms fall into the thick absorption hologram category (Table 1).

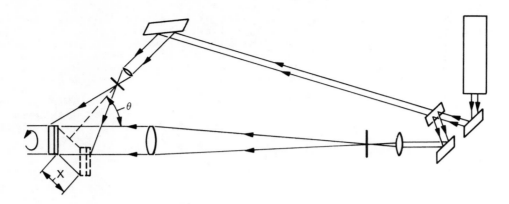

Figure 6.   Optical geometry of construction scanner disk.

Table 1.   Hologram Types and Their Diffraction Efficiency

Hologram Type	Thin		Thick (or Volume)	
	Absorption	Phase	Absorption	Phase
Hologram formed by variation of	Transmittance	Thickness	Transmittance	Refractive Index
Maximum theoretical DE* (%)	6.25	33.9**	3.7	100
Maximum DE* obtained experimentally (%)	--	30**	--	98
Typical recording material	High-resolution photographic films	Photoresist, thermoplastic	High-resolution photographic films	Photopolymer, dichromated gelatin, bleached photo-graphic films

 *DE: Diffraction efficiency
**These DEs are based on sinusoidal modulation.   Properly blazed holograms can produce
   higher DE.

Copying holograms on dichromated gelatin

   Since the achievable diffraction efficiency of thick absorption holograms is typically
2 to 3 percent, these original holograms are not practical.   Therefore, we have developed
techniques for copying the original holographic scanner onto dichromated gelatin plates
to increase the diffraction efficiency.

   Using the processing techniques described in the next section, we successfully made
copies on dichromated gelatin plates derived from Kodak holographic plates, obtaining
diffraction efficiencies as high as 70 percent.   The copying was done by using a
technique similar to photographic contact printing, but at a wavelength of 0.5145 μm.
Since the wvelength (0.5145 μm) used for the copying is different from the wavelength
(0.6328 μm) used for the construction of original holograms, the wavefront used for
copying could not be a plane wave.   The exact waveform of this laser beam can be found
easily by using the Bragg conditions for thick holograms.[16]

   It is possible to increase the diffraction efficiency of copied holograms to more than
90 percent by optimizing the processing steps described in the next section.
Furthermore, if the dichromated gelatin is sensitized for red wavelengths near 0.6328 μm,
the diffraction efficiency of the original holograms can be nearly 100 percent.   Then,
diffraction efficiencies approaching 100 percent may be achieved with hologram copies.

Recording material - dichromated gelatin

There are a number of recording materials for recording either thick or thin phase holograms. These materials include bleached photographic emulsions, dichromated gelatin, photopolymer, photoresist, and thermoplastic. Because of the high diffraction efficiency and signal-to-noise ratio that can be achieved, dichromated gelatin appears to be the best available material for the present fabrication of holographic scanners. The salient features of dichromated gelatin holograms are their large refractive index modulation capacity (even at very high spatial frequencies) and low scattering noise. In addition, dichromated gelatin holograms are clear and colorless; their absorption is thereby very low. The spectral response of this material (unless dye sensitized) is limited to the UV and blue-green regions of the spectrum, however.

Holograms are formed by exposing the dichromated gelatin to an interference pattern of light having a wavelength to which the dichromate is sensitive. In the illuminated regions, the exposure initiates cross-linking between adjacent gelatin molecules. Although the cross-linking itself forms a weak hologram, further processing is required to obtain the large refractive index modulation necessary for the hologram to have high diffraction efficiency. Processing is relatively simple and generally consists of several minutes wash followed by dehydration in one or more isopropanol solutions. The washing step removes the dichromate so that the gelatin is left colorless and insensitive to further exposure. To obtain a large index modulation with low scatter noise, however, it is necessary to control the processing environment and to optimize the post-processing as well as the preprocessing steps.[17]

Preparation of dichromated gelatin layer

Dichromated gelatin layers can be prepared by a number of methods. The simplest procedure begins with the removal of the silver halides and dyes from an unexposed high-resolution photographic emulsion. The gelatin can then be sensitized by soaking in a solution of ammonium dichromate. After drying, it is ready for use. By using a more elaborate procedure that includes a conditioning step prior to sensitization, we obtain holograms characterized by very low scattering noise, better surface quality, and more consistent holographic performance. Tables 2 and 3 show the procedures for Kodak 649F holographic plates.

Although it is convenient to use commercially available photographic emulsions as a source of precoated gelatin layers, it is sometimes necessary or preferable to prepare gelatin layers from solution. This is done, for example, to provide gelatin layers having thicknesses unavailable in commercial photographic emulsions or to permit special substrates such as curved substrates. Standard coating methods include dip coating, doctor blade, and gravity-settling techniques. In dip coating, the method most suitable for curved substrates, the substrate is withdrawn from a gelatin solution at a uniform rate; the substrate retains a thin film of gelatin which has a uniform thickness determined by the solution viscosity and the withdrawal rate. In the doctor blade method, a quantity of coating solution is poured onto the substrate, and a wire or knife blade is drawn across the substrate at a fixed distance from the surface. Relatively thick coatings can be prepared by the gravity-settling technique, in which a carefully measured quantity of solution is poured onto the substrate and allowed to dry slowly with the substrate precisely leveled. Other coating techniques, including spin coating and gelatin transfer, can be used. The coated gelatin layer will be hardened and then sensitized by using procedures similar to those shown in Table 2.

Processing of dichromated gelatin holograms

The method of processing dichromated gelatin holograms as described above is simple and straightforward, but it does not always produce high-quality results. Certain precautions must be observed to prevent formation of opacity on the gelatin surface. Our previous experimental investigations of dichromated gelatin holograms revealed that the saturation refractive index modulation, as well as the thickness of the processed hologram, is greatly affected by the processing environment, especially the relative humidity and temperature in the processing room.

Table 4 presents our standard development procedures for holograms recorded in gelatin layers derived from Kodak 649F plates. With slight modifications, our standard processing techniques shown in Tables 2 and 4 can apply to any type of gelatin layer.

Summary and conclusions

The feasibility of holographic scanners as UPC label readers has been successfully demonstrated by fabricating several multihologram disk scanners which generate lattice scan patterns as shown in Fig. 7. As viewed obliquely here, only the outer circumference

Table 2. Preparation of Dichromated Gelatin Plates

Step	Direction
P-1*	Soak in fixer without hardener for 10 min.
P-2	Wash in running water at 32°C for 5 min; start at 24°C and raise temperature 1.8°C/min to 32°C; following wash, lower temperature at same rate to 24°C.
P-3	Soak in fixer with x hardener (Kodak standard 3.25%) for 10 min.
P-4	Wash in running water for 10 min.
P-5	Rinse in distilled water for 5 min. with agitation.
P-6	Dip into a Photo-Flo 200 solution (1 drop/500 ml) for 30 s and remove the excess with either a photographic sponge or clean wiper blade.
P-7	With plate in horizontal position, dry overnight at room temperature.
	Lighting: Red (dim)
P-8	Soak in x% ammonium-dichromated solution (with 0.x% Photo-Flow 200) for 5 min.
P-9	Wipe ammonium dichromate from glass side of plates.
P-10	With plate in horizontal position, dry overnight at room temperature.

All chemicals are dissolved in distilled water and, except where noted, all steps are at a temperature of 24°C.
For our standard processing, we use 3.125% hardener concentration for Step P-3 and 5% for Step P-8.
*For mixing formulas, see Table 3.

Table 3. Examples of Chemical Mixing Formulas

1. Fixer without hardener: Water, 60 ml; fix concentrate, 20 ml
2. Fixer with x% hardener
   $$x\% = \frac{\text{hardener volume}}{\text{water + concentrate volume}} \times 100\%$$
   a) Kodak fixer with standard hardener (3.125%)
      Water: 60 ml; fix concentrate, 20 ml; Hardener, 2.5 ml
   b) Fixer with 2x hardener (6.25%)
      Water: 60 ml; fix concentrate, 20 ml; Hardener, 5 ml
3. 0.5% ammonium dichromate for development
      Water: 800 ml; ammonium dichromate: 4 g
4. x% ammonium dichromate with 0.x% Photo-Flo
   $$x\% = \frac{\text{ammonium dichromate (g)}}{\text{water (ml)}} \times 100\%$$
   a) 5% ammonium dichromate: 40 g; Photo-Flo: 4 ml
   b) 3% ammonium dichromate: Water: 800 ml; ammonium dichromate: 24 g
      Photo-Flo: 2.4 ml

of the rotating disk is illuminated alternatively by the split laser beams which are impinging on the disk 90° apart. For this feasibility demonstration, we initially recorded holograms at 0.6328 μm in Kodak holographic plates and then copied these holograms into dichromated gelatin plates with a laser beam at 0.5145 μm. The initial holograms are the thick absorption type for which the maximum diffraction efficiency is 3.7 percent, whereas the copied dichromated gelatin holograms are the thick phase type, for which the diffraction efficiency can reach nearly 100 percent. The copying was done by using a simple photographic contact- printing technique, but with a coherent laser beam of 0.5145 μm wavelength for illumination. We observed a diffraction efficiency as high at 70 percent from a copied hologram. If dichromated gelatin is sensitized for red wavelengths near 0.6328 μm, the diffraction efficiency of the original (or master) holograms as well as copied holograms can exceed 95 percent.

The major achievements of this study are:

1. We achieved both spot size and depth of focus requirements necessary for UPC scanners: the average measured spot size of a focused Gaussian laser beam at the limits of the depth of focus was about 248 μm at the $1/e^2$ power points.

Table 4. Standard Development of Dichromated Gelatin Plates

Step	Direction	Lighting
SD-1*	Soak in 0.5 percent solution of ammonium dichromate for 5 min	Red (dim)
SD-2*	Soak in fixer with x percent hardener for 5 min	Red (dim)
SD-3	Wash in running water for 10 min	Room light
SD-4	Dip into a Photo-Flo 200 solution (1 drop/500 ml) 30 s and remove the excess water with photographic sponge	Room light
SD-5	Soak in distilled water for 2 min with agitation	Room light
SD-6	Dehydrate in a 50/50 solution of distilled water and isopropanol for 3 min	Room light
SD-7	Dehydrate in 100 percent isopropanol for 3 min	Room light
SD-8	Free-air dry for at least 1 h	Room light
SD-9	Either bake for 2 h over a hot plate at an elevated temperature, or evaporate residual water in a vacuum chamber	Room light

All chemicals are dissolved in distilled water and, except where noted, all steps are at a temperature of 24°C.
In our standard processing, we use a 3.125 percent hardener concentration for Step SD-2.
*For mixing formulas, see Table 3.

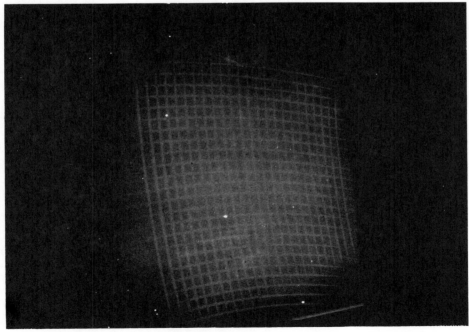

Figure 7. Scan pattern generated by holographic disk.

2. We developed a copying technique and modified processing techniques for copied dichromated gelatin holograms, obtaining high-quality holograms having diffraction efficiency.
3. We designed several optical configurations capable of generating high-density lattice scanning or radial offset scanning patterns, as shown in Fig. 8 through Fig. 11. Based on our analyses, these schemes are cost-effective and suitable for commercial bar code applications.

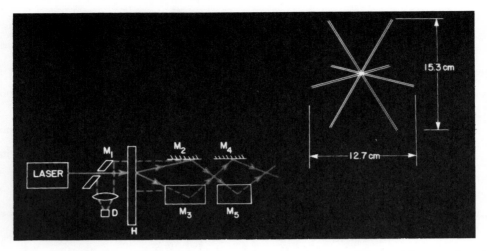

Figure 8. Single beam/off-set hologram scanning configuration and pattern.

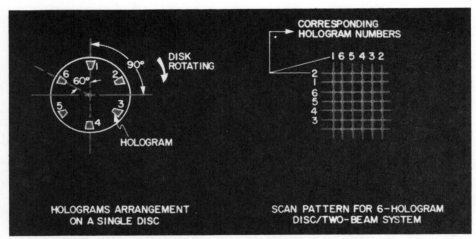

Figure 9. A high-density scan pattern generation.

Acknowledgments

This work was performed while the author was with the Advanced Development Department of NCR Corporation, Cambridge Facility. The author expresses appreciation to Drs. B. Chang and I. Cindrich of ERIM for many valuable discussions and technical assistance. The author also wishes to thank Drs. J. Thunen and T. Zaccone of the Optical Sciences Department, Research & Development Division, Lockheed Missiles & Space Company, Inc. for their encouragement and assistance in many ways that enabled this paper to be presented and published.

References

1. "Scanning Installation Up-date," Food Market Institute, Inc., Washington, D.C., (Dec 1985).

2. C. K. Cheng, "Laser Scanning for UPC Symbols," Proc. Electro-Optical Systems Design Conf., New York, N.Y., (Sep 1976).

3. I. Cindrich, "Image Scanning by Rotation of a Hologram," Appl. Opt. 6, 1531 (1967).

4. D. H. McMahon, A. R. Franklin, and J. B. Thaxter, "Light Beam Deflection Using Holographic Scanning Techniques," Appl. Opt. 8, 399 (1969).

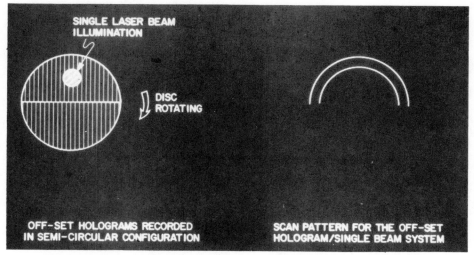

Figure 10. An off-set hologram scanning configuration.

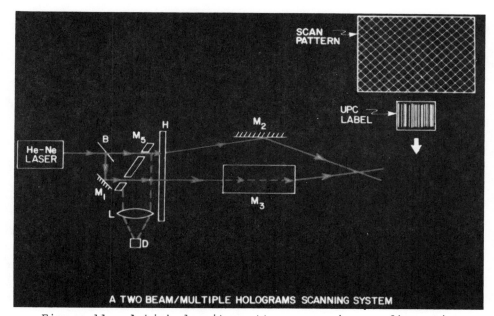

Figure 11. A high-density pattern scanning configuration.

5. L. Beiser et al., "Holofacet Laser Scanning," Proc. Electro-Optical Systems Design Conf. (Sep 1973).

6. R. V. Pole and H. W. Wallenman, "Holographic Laser Beam Deflector," Appl. Opt. 14, 976 (1976).

7. J. C. Wyant, "Rotating Diffraction Grating Laser Beam Scanner," Appl. Opt. 14, 1057 (1975).

8. O. Bryngdahl and W. Lee, "Laser Beam Scanning Using Computer-Generated Holograms," Appl. Opt. 15, 183 (1976).

9. C. S. Ih, "Holographic Laser Beam Scanners Utilizing an Auxiliary Reflector," Appl. Opt. 16, 2137 (1977).

10. L. Beiser, U.S. Patent 3,614,193 (1971); Electro-Opt. Syst. Des. 33 (Oct 1973).

11. A. Bramley, U.S. Patent 3,721,486 (1973); Appl. Opt. $\underline{8}$, 2780 (1973).

12. G. Pieuchard, J. Glamand, and A. Labeyrie, U.S. Patent 3,721,487 (1973).

13. C. K. Cheng, U. S. Patent 4,224,509 (1981).

14. E. B. Champagne, "A Qualitative and Quantitative Study of Holographic Imaging," Technical Report AFAL-TR-67-107 (July 1967).

15. J. N. Latta, "Computer-Based Analysis of Hologram Imagery and Aberrations, I. Hologram Types and their Nonchromatic Aberrations," Appl. Opt. $\underline{10}$, 599 (1971).

16. H. Kogelnik, "Coupled Wave Theory for Thick Hologram Gratings," The Bell System Technical Journal $\underline{48}$, 2909 (1969).

17. B. J. Chang and C. Leonard, "Exposure Characteristics of Dichromated Gelatin Holograms," presented at the October 1976 Annual Meeting of the Optical Society of America, Tucson, AZ.

AUTHOR INDEX